THE**FOOD**DOCTOR
DIET
CLUB

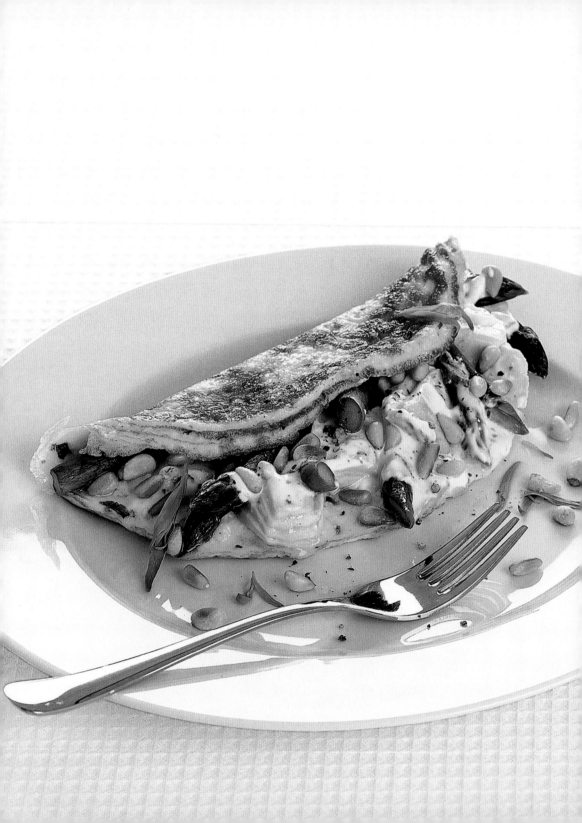

THE FOODDOCTOR
DIET CLUB

Ian Marber Dip ION

Recipes by Rowena Paxton Dip ION

To join The Food Doctor Diet Club visit
www.thefooddoctor.com

LONDON, NEW YORK, MELBOURNE, MUNICH AND DELHI

For Trish, the best friend anyone could wish for

Project editor Susannah Steel
Project designer Jo Grey
Senior editor Shannon Beatty
Senior art editor Anne Fisher
Managing editor Penny Warren
Managing art editor Marianne Markham
Publishing operations manager Gillian Roberts
DTP designer Sonia Charbonnier
Production controller Luca Frassinetti
Creative publisher Mary-Clare Jerram
Art director Peter Luff
Food stylists Jo Pratt, Sarah Tildesley
Photography of food Sîan Irvine
Photography of Ian Marber and Diet Club members Francis Loney

First published in Great Britain in 2007 by
Dorling Kindersley Limited,
80 Strand, London WC2R 0RL

A Penguin Company

2 4 6 8 10 9 7 5 3

A CIP catalogue record for this book is available from the British Library

ISBN 978-1-4053-1690-3

Colour reproduced by Colourscan, Singapore
Printed and bound in China by Leo Paper Products Ltd

Discover more at
www.dk.com

Contents

Analyzing your lifestyle

Week 1: fresh start

Weeks 2 & 3: readjusting

Week 4 & beyond: eat better forever

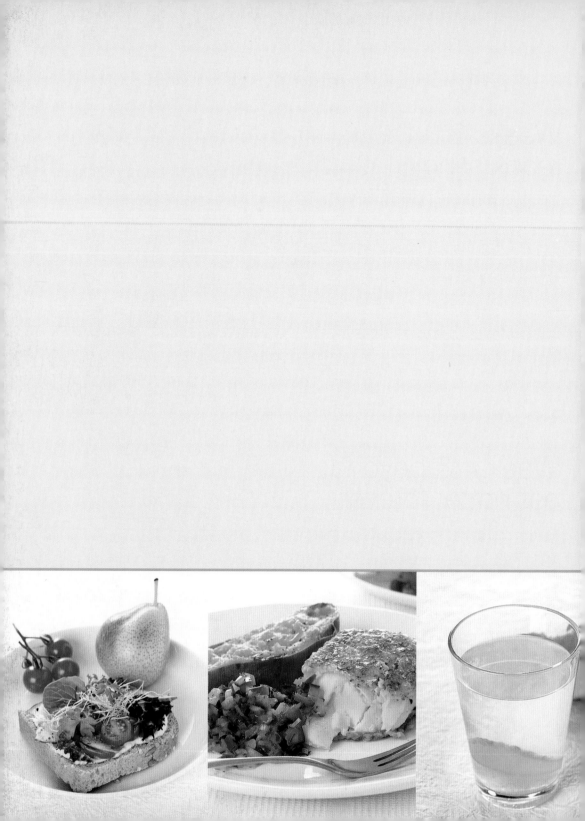

Analyzing your lifestyle

We all like to feel that we are healthy and eating well, but how much do you really understand about the way that food converts into energy, and the biochemistry that dictates how well you feel, as well as how much you weigh? This chapter will test your knowledge and give you the basics on eating well.

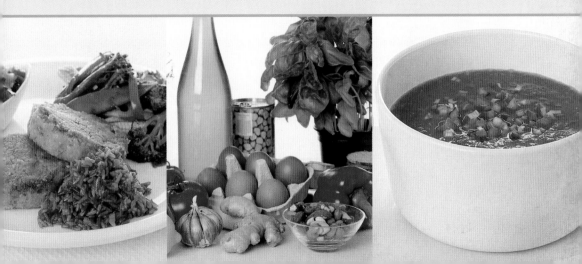

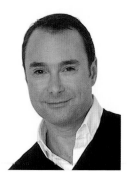

Introduction

In this age of diet-related health issues and celebrity obsession, we are all under pressure to "eat well". It's the driving force that motivates millions of us to look at what we're eating.

The greatest problem we face when it comes to weight issues is how to sort out the truth from information and advice that is commercially driven. Newspapers are full of features about weight loss, miracle nutrients, scientific breakthroughs and food labelling. They also carry horror stories of diet-related diseases and shortened life spans. Despite all this, we don't seem to make changes to our diet until we feel pressured to lose weight.

Social pressure

If you do eat well, then surely the outward manifestation of that is being slim, isn't it? I feel that the influence of social pressure goes further than that: if people are slim, we believe that they are "good", in control of their lives and thus to be admired. In our society, that's a mark of success.

Conversely, if you are overweight, does this signify that you are a bad person, out of control, to be scorned and pitied?

So what about the vast majority of us who try to eat well, or have dieted forever, but simply can't lose weight unless we eat next to nothing and exercise furiously? The millions of people who have battled with their weight for years – or even those of us who aren't obese, but feel we should just be a little slimmer – are understandably influenced by the pressure generated by the marketing and media aspects of the food industry.

It is always distressing to see people in my clinic whose feelings of self worth are directly tied in to what they weigh. To them, fat is bad, slim is good, and they experience these thoughts at some level every day. Therefore, when the next diet or wonder food is trumpeted, it's entirely understandable that they will leap at it, even if the diet may go against their natural instincts.

The diet treadmill

Imagine a business that had to create something new every single day, without exception, and present new ideas and products to its customers accordingly. If it didn't, it would risk losing the customers to a rival who is offering them what they want. That's what marketing and the media, in all its forms, constantly have to do. We buy magazines, read features, follow the diets, lose weight. If a diet is too successful, other publications will investigate how safe it is and bring any doubts about the diet to their readers' attention – and so another media source brings its influence to bear on what we think. This leaves us wanting a replacement for that diet and, sure enough, there is bound to be one. And if the media can attach a celebrity to a new diet, so much the better.

This constant bombardment of potentially conflicting information confuses the issues. Add in the social pressures to be slim and, all of a sudden, anyone who wants to lose weight just doesn't know what to eat anymore.

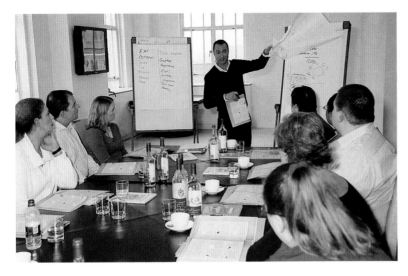

Telling it as it is
My job is to explain the basic science behind what happens to food after you eat it so that you can make better food choices.

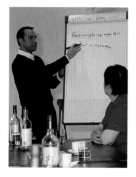

Confusing **information** and social **pressures** mean we **don't** know what **to eat** anymore if we want to **lose weight**

Marketing tactics

Food manufacturers and supermarkets have a duty of care to their shareholders to maximize profits and minimize costs. Some trade ethically, others less so, but still within the letter of the law (especially when it comes to food labelling).

These days, we are told that we lead very busy lives and are too busy to cook for ourselves, so we can now buy ready meals and snacks that the food industry terms "meal solutions". This is ironic, as one could argue that it's convenience foods that have partially created the "meal problem" in the first place. The marketing and labels are cleverly presented to appeal not only to the time-poor, but also to those of us who want fresh food that won't add to any weight problems. Better still, if the food has an aura of aiding weight loss, it has an increased value to us and we buy it more often. Take a moment to reflect on the ready foods you buy – diet or otherwise – which you could actually make yourself for next to nothing. I have found that even my busiest clients can make time to prepare simple, basic meals and snacks that form the foundation of a successful food plan.

Our metabolic rate

With all that in mind, how does The Food Doctor Diet differ? My plan works because you gain a healthy understanding of the real value of food and eat regularly; other diets ultimately fail because they are about deprivation. But what does this mean in terms of how our bodies work?

I believe that our lifestyles and history of dieting (be it in the extreme, or just too frequently) affect our metabolic rate, so any initial success at weight loss will be followed by a natural physiological response in our bodies: as our inbuilt metabolic rate senses famine, the weight loss slows or stops. We feel we must be doing something wrong, blame ourselves, and perpetuate any feelings of low self-worth we may have. We try harder by eating a little less or exercising a little harder, and thus trying to cheat our metabolism. It can't be done, but we are influenced to such a degree that we feel it can. So, it's back on the diet treadmill again – though, in the long run, we lose everything except the weight.

The science of energy

Energy cannot be created or destroyed; it merely changes its state. This is the basic law of energy. Thus the food we eat becomes glucose, which is used as fuel to make energy, and if our cells make full use of that glucose, no energy is changed into fat. It seems logical that if you eat more than you need, the surplus will be stored as fat and, conversely, eating less will force stored fat to be released. In practice, this doesn't always work as planned because of how we think and feel (our desires and goals cannot be separated from our physiology) and because of the numerous influences on our metabolism. Our metabolism dictates the speed at which we function. If you imagine this in terms of a car, its "metabolism" is a combination of the size of the car, the engine and the availability and quality of the fuel used.

Storing and releasing energy

When glucose levels in the blood exceed the body's needs (due to the amount of food we eat), they are first stored away in a water-based solution called glycogen. If glucose requirements increase, glycogen is released to meet the need and the water in which it was held is excreted. This reduction in hydration is one of the reasons why we lose weight quickly and urinate more when

My plan **works** because you gain a **healthy** understanding of the **real value** of food and **eat regularly**

we first start a diet that does not provide optimum levels of fuel from food. In order to succeed with The Food Doctor Diet plan, we need to have a good understanding of some basic truths. So, a reduction in energy intake (i.e., food) will result in weight loss. The problem is that we don't cut our intake by, say, five per cent: offered the choice of a diet that could enable you to lose excess weight – say, two stone (12.7kg) – in a year, or one that promises the same results in two months, which one would you go for? If you are someone who has battled with weight issues for many years, then it's natural that you'd want to try the quickest diet.

When we take in too few calories, or expend too much energy, many things occur. If we eat too little, which is the only way that quick weight-loss promises can be fulfilled, then we alert our metabolic rate to potential or likely famine, and it begins to behave accordingly. It will slow down the release of fat and trigger the adrenal glands *(below)* to produce energy to make up the shortfall. However, we need a certain amount of energy to help us move around, so if you are a particular size, eating too little results in energy having to be released from elsewhere in the body to meet energy requirements. Fat isn't always the first choice as it's not easy to break down, and I have found that it is often people's adrenaline levels that increase instead.

Glucose-raising agents (GRA)

Bear in mind that it's not just eating food that raises our glucose levels. When we encounter stress, the adrenal glands are stimulated to secrete adrenaline, which may temporarily provide us with the energy we need to react to the situation. It's like the battery in the car, providing a separate source of energy that works independently of fuel levels. As there are countless stress triggers

In order to **succeed** with The Food Doctor Diet plan, we **need** to have a **good** understanding of some **basic truths**

Adrenaline is a **wild card** and we **cannot** regulate it in the **same** way as we do with **food**

in modern life, this reaction is frequent, and it is common for the adrenal glands to be over-stimulated. Think of the mornings when you haven't eaten, but feel energetic and capable; by rights, you should feel tired and lethargic. Adrenaline is a wild card and we can't regulate it like we do with food.

Fat cells do not give up their contents easily: if we have too much adrenaline, our energy requirements are met, so the fat cells can often take this as a sign to stop releasing their stores. If the process of fat being released to be converted back into glucose is hindered or even halted by adrenaline being released, the total energy intake is now in excess of 100 per cent, so some of the food we eat must be stored as fat. Until the signal for the adrenal glands is switched off, this situation can perpetuate. The problem is that the signal isn't always reliable, as adrenal glands can become overly responsive due to almost constant stimuli. A major trigger of adrenaline is a result of low levels of glucose in the blood – something that can be regulated on The Food Doctor Diet plan.

Caffeine also provides short-term energy by blocking the action of a chemical called adensine in the brain. The pituitary gland senses a problem and tells the adrenal glands to secrete adrenaline to combat this block, leading to excess glucose and a subsequent low in energy levels.

So if you eat too little, are anxious or stressed or drink excess amounts of caffeine, you no longer lose weight. You then eat even less – and end up feeling fatigued, denying yourself food, developing cravings, and perpetuating metabolic issues: the moment you cut your calorie intake, you cut your metabolic rate. Thus the metabolism slows down into famine mode and tries to hold on to its fat.

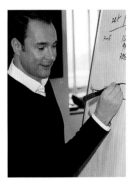

Aside from the issue of **weight loss**, my **Food Doctor plan** will **benefit** you in ways that most diets cannot **match**

How to eat well

The Food Doctor Diet plan minimizes the influence that GRAs create in several ways. Firstly, food groups are combined in the right proportions. When eaten alone, carbohydrates such as bread and potatoes are like a thin, runny fuel, which is converted into energy quickly. However, this energy runs out equally quickly, so we need to eat sooner. (If you're dieting and eating mainly carbohydrates, you apply willpower because you don't want to eat too much food, possibly triggering an adrenaline release.)

Complex carbohydrates create the equivalent of a thicker liquid, as they have a higher content of fibre that is harder to break down. Eaten alone, however, even complex carbohydrates are potentially too available (that is, too runny), so the energy is used relatively quickly and we feel hungry again. The simple addition of protein and fat at every meal means that the energy produced is like a thick and gooey fuel, so it's released in a measured way. This gives steady glucose levels to feed cells evenly, and we have sufficient energy until the next intake of food.

Secondly, portion size is vital: eating the perfect amount of food in the right proportions to create the glucose we need – no more than that – and then eating again within three hours starts the process of retraining the metabolism to understand that you

Why other diets fail

REDUCED CALORIE INTAKE	= Less energy released, disrupted metabolic rate, raised adrenaline levels
RESULT	= Unsustainable diet regime, fatigue, hunger cravings, slow or no further weight loss

Why The Food Doctor Diet works

SMALL REGULAR MEALS = Energy released consistently, active
metabolic rate, reduced need for adrenaline

RESULT = High energy levels, no hunger cravings,
steady weight loss

are in a time of just enough and not too much, and certainly not too little to trigger the famine mode. In short, you take in fuel in the morning, use it up, re-fuel mid-morning and again at lunch, snack time and lastly at dinner. Frequent, consistent meals of the ideal ratio and size will trigger weight loss that can be sustained. This is an essential part of The Food Doctor Diet plan.

Thirdly, using fresh food with maximum nutrient content means that you'll have a decreased risk of common diseases, better sleep and digestion and more energy. Lots of other things will change too, and not necessarily what you'd expect: you'll have better skin, hair and nails, your moods will improve and you will feel more in control of what and how to eat.

My plan is 30 days long: two days of preparation and four weeks of carefully structured menu plans and recipes. You'll avoid sugar, red meat and alcohol for the month, so don't be tempted to go to too many restaurants or parties if you want to ensure success. Preparation is all-important: read ahead, know what you're doing and shop for the necessary foods beforehand. Preparation day 1 begins on a Tuesday, and weeks 1–4 start on successive Thursdays.

The truth is simple, and it works. Aside from the obvious issue of weight loss, my plan will benefit you in ways that most diets cannot match: you'll regulate your metabolic rate; you won't worry about passing fads; you'll eat well forever and never feel deprived; and you'll be in the best of health. Good luck!

Questionnaire

Use this questionnaire to see how your diet and lifestyle currently affect your well-being. Note down your score for each question, add up all the scores and assess your results on page 19.

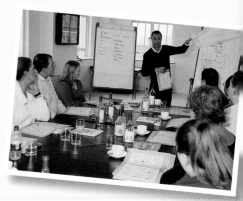

HEALTH CONDITIONS

DIGESTION

How often do you suffer from the following?	A Frequently	B Sometimes	C Rarely	D Never
Belching/wind/flatulence	4	3	2	1
Abdominal bloating	4	③	2	1
Indigestion	4	3	②	1
White-coated tongue	4	3	②	1
Diarrhoea or loose stools	4	3	②	1
Constipation/straining to pass stools	4	3	②	1
Bad breath	4	③	2	1
Upset stomach	4	3	②	1

SCORE [ ]

BLOOD SUGAR MANAGEMENT

How often do you suffer from the following?	A Frequently	B Sometimes	C Rarely	D Never
Need to eat meals or snacks regularly	④	3	2	1
Need coffee/tea/cigarettes	4	3	②	1
Drowsiness or extreme fatigue during the day	④	3	2	1
Need more than 8 hours sleep a night	4	③	2	1
Slow to wake in the morning	④	3	2	1
Dizziness or irritability without food	④	3	2	1

	A	B	C	D
	Frequently	Sometimes	Rarely	Never
Loss of concentration if you miss a meal	(4)	3	2	1
Have sweet or starchy food cravings	(4)	3	2	1
Cravings for alcohol	4	3	2	(1)
Mood swings	4	(3)	2	1

SCORE **33**

FEMALE HEALTH

How often do you suffer from the following?	A	B	C	D
	Frequently	Sometimes	Rarely	Never
Breast tenderness or water retention	4	(3)	2	1
Low libido	4	(3)	2	1

SCORE **6**

MALE HEALTH

How often do you suffer from the following?	A	B	C	D
	Frequently	Sometimes	Rarely	Never
Loss of motivation and drive	4	3	2	1
Low libido	4	3	2	1

SCORE

METABOLISM

How often do you suffer from the following?	A	B	C	D
	Frequently	Sometimes	Rarely	Never
Hair loss on head or outer third of eyebrows	4	(3)	2	1
Sensitivity to the cold	4	(3)	2	1
Ongoing fatigue	4	3	(2)	1
Difficulty with weight loss	(4)	3	2	1
Dry or scaly skin	(4)	3	2	1

SCORE **16**

DIET AND LIFESTYLE

HOW GOOD IS YOUR CURRENT DIET?

How often do you eat/drink the following?	A Every day	B Every week	C Rarely	D Never
Sugary snacks (chocolate, biscuits, sweets, cakes)	(4)	3	2	1
Sugar in tea, coffee or cereals	4	3	2	(1)
Cans of fizzy drink (including energy drinks)	4	3	(2)	1
White bread, pasta, white rice	4	3	(2)	1
Shallow- or deep-fried foods	4	3	(2)	1
Tea and coffee	(4)	3	2	1
Alcohol	4	3	2	(1)
Red meat	4	3	(2)	1
Processed foods and ready meals	4	3	2	(1)
Takeaway food	4	(3)	2	1

SCORE 22

How often do you eat/drink the following?	A Every day	B Every week	C Rarely	D Never
3 pieces of fresh fruit	(1)	2	3	4
2 portions of fresh vegetables	(1)	2	3	4
Oily fish (sardines, mackerel, etc)	1	2	(3)	4
Seeds (pumpkin seeds, sunflower seeds, etc)	1	(2)	3	4
Raw unsalted/roasted nuts	(1)	2	3	4
Wholegrains (brown bread, rice and pasta, etc)	(1)	2	3	4
Bean and pulses (chickpeas, lentils, kidney beans, etc)	1	(2)	3	4
8 glasses of bottled or filtered water	(1)	2	3	4
Lean protein (chicken, turkey, tofu, etc)	(1)	2	3	4
Raw food (salad, raw vegetables, etc)	1	(2)	3	4

SCORE 15

EXERCISE

Do you do the following?	A Always	B Sometimes	C Rarely	D Never
Take cardiovascular exercise at least 3 times per week	(1)	2	3	4
Walk for more than 20 mins a day	1	2	3	(4)

SCORE 5

FINAL SCORE

Mostly As or a score of 142–188

This score indicates that there is a lot that you can do to improve your overall health and wellness. It is likely that there are a number of factors that could be contributing towards your inability to lose weight (or the fact that you have been gaining weight). It is important that you focus on improving your overall digestive health and address any issues that may have to do with blood sugar imbalance. The Food Doctor Diet Club plan will help to give you a kick-start by eliminating the blood sugar highs you're having and re-educating you as to the right foods to eat.

Mostly Bs or a score of 95–141

There are still a number of things that you could do to make your diet better. You need to replace processed foods or ready meals with fresh foods where possible and start preparing your own meals. The Food Doctor Diet Club plan will give you the guidance and confidence you need to prepare your own healthy meals, improve your well-being and lose weight.

Mostly Cs or a score of 47–94

This score indicates that your overall health and wellness seem to be in good shape. It is likely that you do not have any underlying digestive problems and that you are eating in a way that leads to consistent energy levels. Generally you are making good food choices, but The Food Doctor Diet Club plan will help you incorporate The Food Doctor principles (pp.136–37) into your diet so that you'll feel your best.

"Lots of symptoms should noticeably improve or disappear when you follow my plan"

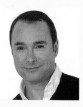

10 pre-plan Diet Club members

Our 10 participants have chosen to follow The Food Doctor Diet Club plan for many different reasons. The one thing they all have in common is that they want to lose weight and develop a more positive attitude towards eating. Here they introduce themselves, giving some reasons why they've joined the club and how they're feeling.

Mary

Age 48
Height 1.74m (5ft 8½in)
Weight 84kg (13st 3lb)
Dress size 16
Occupation Pilates teacher

Despite dieting since I was 20 years old, I've never been successful at achieving a weight I'm comfortable with. I still see food as a means of reward or comfort. I want to change the ingredients I use and the way I prepare them so that the whole family can all eat healthily. I also need to begin a healthy eating plan to help me cope with the effects of the menopause. I'm apprehensive about starting The Food Doctor Diet Club plan, as controlling my eating is something I have always failed at and I don't want to fail again.

"I can't control what I eat"

Silvia

Age 39
Height 1.72m (5ft 8in)
Weight 95kg (14st 13lb)
Dress size 18
Occupation Production manager

I'm the mother of a two-year-old girl. Since the birth of my daughter I've been trying to lose weight, but with no success. My problem is that I need someone to direct me and advise me on what I should be eating, and the quantities I should be having. I feel quite excited and positive about starting The Food Doctor Diet Club plan, but I'm a bit apprehensive about the amount of new meals I will be cooking, and I will miss eating chocolate.

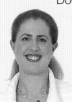

"I've been trying to lose weight since my daughter's birth"

Brendan

Age 30
Height 1.88m (6ft 2in)
Weight 98kg (15st 6lb)
Waist 97cm (38in)
Occupation Graphic designer

I have just hit 30, and I'm developing a worryingly avocado-like figure. I also have slightly high blood pressure, which is something I need to keep an eye on. I am enrolled at a gym, but the only pounds I seem to be losing are those from my wallet. I don't think I eat badly, but I know I eat at the wrong times. I need a bit of help and guidance to get my body back into the correct age bracket!

"I have high blood pressure"

Rachael

Age 30
Height 1.59m (5ft 2½in)
Weight 137kg (21st 7lb)
Dress size 28/30 (top/bottom)
Occupation Senior administrator

I suffer from recurrent colds and headaches, and also from poor concentration, which I'm sure has something to do with the kinds of food I eat. I really need to lose weight and get fit. A couple of years ago I had a real scare: after the birth of my second child I had a pulmonary embolism (PE) and almost died. I need to improve my chances of not having another PE. I have two lovely children and a devoted husband and I want to be around for them more than ever now. I want my son to bring his friends home and hear them say, "Wow, your mum's fit!"

"I want to be around for my family more than ever now"

Lynne

Age 53
Height 1.70m (5ft 7in)
Weight 76kg (12st 3lb)
Dress size 14/16 (top/bottom)
Occupation Personal assistant

I've given up smoking, and the last time I did this I piled on nearly 9.5 kilograms (1½ stone). I am not very good at dieting, but I am a miserable 12.7 kilograms (2 stone) heavier than I should be, and my GP has advised that I lose this weight before I have an operation later on this year. I want to feel fitter, and I know that losing weight will help, but my willpower is very poor and I need encouragement to keep at it.

"I've given up smoking and don't want to put on weight"

Jon

Age 36
Height 1.88m (6ft 2in)
Weight 139kg (21st 12lb)
Waist 130cm (51in)
Occupation Signals operations manager

Joan

Age 32
Height 1.68m (5ft 6in)
Weight 95kg (14st 13lb)
Dress size 22/20 (top/bottom)
Occupation Buying assistant

We've both tried other diets before, but they haven't worked. We tried Weight Watchers and spent all day thinking about food and points, and we did the Atkins Diet. Our weakness was takeaways. We want to have children and we both need to lose weight to improve our chances. Jon also has high blood pressure and cholesterol and works shifts, including nights. Eating healthily needs to become a priority for us.

Jon: I feel quite nervous, and yet excited as well, about going on the plan. I'm really hoping that this won't be one of those diets that works for a short while and then I'll return to my normal eating habits and put on weight again. I'm very worried about giving up tea as I drink so much of it.

Joan: I'm feeling quite happy about starting The Food Doctor plan. I'm not looking forward to giving up fast food, chocolate or vodka, but I'll cope.

"Eating healthily needs to be a priority for both of us"

Katie

Age 27
Height 1.77m (5ft 10in)
Weight 82.1kg (12st 13lb)
Dress size 18/20 (top/bottom)
Occupation Cartographer

In the last six months I've lost 3.2 kilograms (½ stone) by eating recipes from a Weight Watchers diet book, but I haven't followed it strictly and I haven't lost any more weight. Most of this weight has been lost from just my legs rather than from the top half of my body too. I'm looking forward to trying the new foods on The Food Doctor Diet Club plan, but I'm going to find it hard to give up red meat and tea – I usually have about six to 10 cups of tea a day.

"I can't lose any more weight"

Chris

Age 43
Height 1.80m (5ft 11in)
Weight 91.3kg (14st 5lb)
Waist 86cm (34in)
Occupation Life coach and hypnotherapist

I have acid stomach problems, and I regularly take medication for gastro oesophageal reflux disease (GORD). I want to be able to keep this condition under control. I also want to improve my energy levels and reach the recommended medical weight for my height. I'm looking forward to shedding some weight, but I'm a little apprehensive because I have a busy job and I'm time-poor. I'm expecting I'll miss my cups of tea and my morning cappuccino.

"I want to improve my energy levels"

Karen

Age 47
Height 1.70m (5ft 7in)
Weight 93kg (14st 8lb)
Dress size 20
Occupation Analyst/programmer

I'm about 25–32 kilograms (4–5 stone) overweight. I work in IT and have a totally sedentary job. I get very little exercise and I eat too much – usually many of the wrong things. I'm looking for a new way of approaching food, rather than a quick weight-loss programme (I've tried many of those and failed). I have the reassuring feeling that this is a "gourmet diet". I've been to slimming clubs in the past, looked at the menus and worried that there's nothing I would normally eat. I'm feeling very positive about this plan.

"i'm looking for a new way of approaching food"

Your view

Like all these participants preparing to begin The Food Doctor Diet Club plan, it's worth you taking a moment to analyze where you have gone wrong in the past, and what it is that you are keen to change about your eating habits.

Pre-plan food diary

Before you begin The Food Doctor 30-day Diet plan, keep a food diary of what you eat and drink over the next three days. This will help you to identify which foods presently make up the bulk of your usual diet, and to clarify the current state of your health *(see also pp.16–19)*. It will also be interesting for you to look back after you finish the plan and see how differently you ate.

Accurate accounts

To record an accurate diary, you should include all drinks, snacks and meals, and the time you had them. You should also make a note of how you feel during, and at the end of, each day. Make sure you don't leave anything out: although this is for your reference only, it will help you to understand why you feel like you do now when you compare your results at the end of the plan.

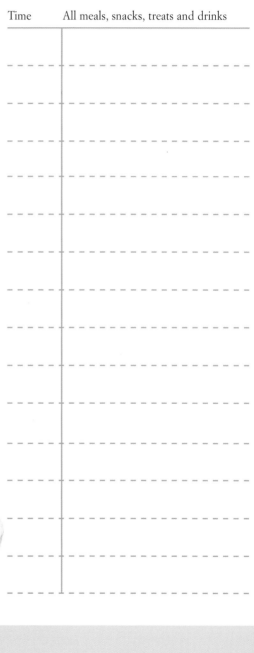

FIRST DAY

Time	All meals, snacks, treats and drinks

SECOND DAY

Time	All meals, snacks, treats and drinks

THIRD DAY

Time	All meals, snacks, treats and drinks

Shopping list for days 1 & 2 & soup recipes

This list is repeated at the back of the book: just rip out page 181 to take shopping with you. Use this list to check for any items you may already have.

Fruit
- [ ] Apples, 4
- [ ] Bananas, 1
- [ ] Lemons, 2
- [ ] Limes, 1
- [ ] Pears, 1

Vegetables
- [ ] Carrots, approx. 50g (2oz)
- [ ] Cherry tomatoes, 1 tub
- [ ] Cucumbers, small, 2
- [ ] Mixed raw vegetables, approx. 600g (1lb 3½oz)
- [ ] Mixed salad ingredients: enough for 2 portions
- [ ] Onions, medium, 1
- [ ] Onions, small, 2
- [ ] Peppers, green, 1
- [ ] Peppers, red, 1
- [ ] Red onion, small, 1
- [ ] Spring onions, 1 bunch
- [ ] Sweet potatoes, large, 1
- [ ] Tomatoes, medium, 2

Fresh herbs
- [ ] Basil, fresh, 1 packet
- [ ] Parsley, fresh, 1 bunch

Dairy
- [ ] Hen's eggs, 1
- [ ] Live natural low-fat yoghurt, 1 large pot

- [ ] Haloumi, 200g (7oz) (if making Oat-crumb haloumi, day 2)
- [ ] Orange or apple juice, 1 carton
- [ ] Peppermint tea, 1 packet
- [ ] Oatcakes, 1 packet

Meat & fish
- [ ] Beef mince, very lean, 200g (7oz) (if making Beef burgers, day 1)
- [ ] White fish fillet (cod, haddock etc.), 200g (7oz), (if making Oat-crumb fish, day 2)

Storecupboard foods
- [ ] *Chick-peas, 1x400g (13oz) can (if making Chick-pea burgers, day 1)
- [ ] Oat flakes, 1 packet
- [ ] Rice, Camargue (red) or brown, 1 packet
- [ ] Mixed seeds, 1 tub (or see p.51)
- [ ] Nuts, raw unsalted, 1 small packet

Spices & flavourings
- [ ] Chilli powder, 1 small jar
- [ ] Cumin powder, 1 small jar
- [ ] Herbes de Provence, 1 pot

- [ ] Mustard, 1 small pot
- [ ] Olive oil, 1 bottle
- [ ] Soy sauce, 1 bottle
- [ ] Stock, vegetable, 150ml (¼ pint) or yeast-free bouillon powder, 1 tub

FOR THE WINTER SOUPS
(Carrot, leek & watercress soup, Tomato & mixed vegetable soup)
- [ ] Carrots, 500g (1lb 2oz)
- [ ] Celery, 1 bunch
- [ ] Garlic bulbs, 1
- [ ] Leeks, medium, 1
- [ ] Onions, medium, 1
- [ ] Onions, small, 1
- [ ] Red pepper, large, 1
- [ ] Watercress, fresh, 2 bunches
- [ ] *Cannellini beans, 1x400g (13oz) can
- [ ] *Chick-peas, 1x400g (13oz) can
- [ ] Plum tomatoes, chopped, 1x400g (13oz) can
- [ ] Basil (dried), 1 small jar
- [ ] Mango powder, 1 small jar
- [ ] Smoked paprika, 1 jar
- [ ] Vegetable stock, 2 litres (3½ pints) or yeast-free bouillon powder, 1 tub (if not bought for prep days)

FOR THE SUMMER SOUPS

(Light vegetable broth, Chilled summer soup)

- [ ] Lemons, 2
- [ ] Baby corn, 100g (3½oz)
- [ ] Carrots, 100g (3½oz)
- [ ] Cucumber, ½
- [ ] Baby leeks 100g (3½oz) or spring onions, 1 bunch
- [ ] Mangetout, 100g (3½oz)
- [ ] Pepper, 1 (any colour)

- [ ] Red onion, medium, 1
- [ ] Root ginger, fresh, 1 piece
- [ ] Fresh coriander, 1 bunch
- [ ] Apple juice, 1 carton
- [ ] Vegetable juice, 1 carton
- [ ] *Cannellini beans, 1x400g (13oz) can
- [ ] Plum tomatoes, chopped, 1x400g (13oz) can

- [ ] Miso paste, 1 packet
- [ ] Quinoa, 1 packet
- [ ] Tomato purée, 1 tube
- [ ] Tabasco, 1 bottle
- [ ] Vegetable stock (good quality) to make 1.6 litres (2¾ pints) or yeast-free bouillon powder, 1 tub (if not bought for prep days)

*All cans should be free from added salt and sugar

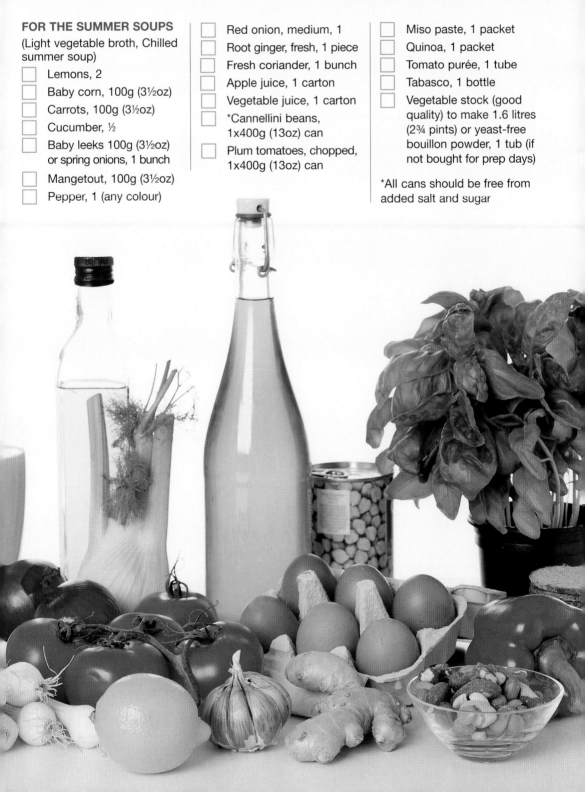

preparing for the plan
days 1-2

Breakfast

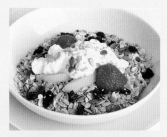

Have your usual cereal, but add 1 tablespoon of live natural low-fat yoghurt and some fresh fruit.

Dilute juice with water for a 50:50 mix. Avoid caffeine.

Morning snack

Orange or apple juice diluted 50:50 with water, or a cup of peppermint tea.

If you usually eat biscuits around this time of day, eat 1 tablespoon of pumpkin seeds too.

Lunch

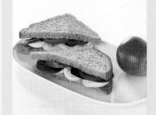

Have 3–4 cherry tomatoes and an apple with your sandwiches or lunchtime meal.

Breakfast

50g (2oz) of your usual cereal with 1 tablespoon of pumpkin seeds, 1 chopped apple and 1 tablespoon live natural low-fat yoghurt.

Drink diluted juice or herb tea. Avoid caffeine.

Morning snack

Diluted juice or herb tea with 12 mixed raw nuts or ½ banana and 1 oatcake.

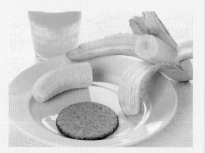

Lunch

Take away the top layer of your sandwiches and have it with 4 tomatoes. Eat either a pear or an apple with your lunch.

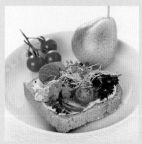

Tip for the day ...

When you shop, look out for varieties of flavoured seed mixes on sale, as they make a tasty alternative to plain seeds.

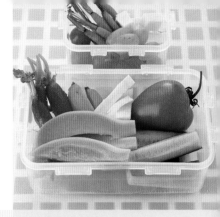

Afternoon snack

Diluted juice or tea or coffee made weaker than you usually have it and without sugar.

If you normally eat sweet biscuits, have ½ banana and 1 tablespoon of pumpkin seeds instead.

Dinner

Home-made beef or chick-pea burgers with red rice & stir-fried vegetables *(p.32)*.

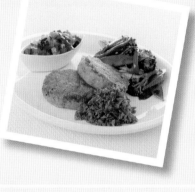

Afternoon snack

Diluted juice or herb tea with 2 oatcakes, ½ banana or 1 apple and 1 tablespoon of pumpkin seeds.

Dinner

Oat-crumbed fish fillet or haloumi with baked sweet potato & mixed salad *(p.33)*.

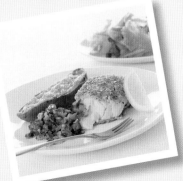

Foods to enjoy

Vegetables in as many different colours as possible, apples, pears, cherries, berries, lemons, limes, any other fruit in moderation, avocados, oats, quinoa, millet, rye, brown, red or wild rice, seeds, nuts in moderation, organic eggs, organic chicken, turkey, fish, tofu, unprocessed cheese such as goat's cheese, herb teas, herbs and spices.

Make your own sprouted seeds now to enjoy while you are on the plan. See page 151 to find out how.

Foods to avoid

Tea, coffee, fizzy drinks, alcohol, undiluted fruit juice, salted snacks, crisps, sweet biscuits, cakes, confectionery, ice cream, white bread, white pasta, white rice, potatoes, most commercial cereals, processed cheese, flavoured yoghurts, fried foods, bacon, red meat, sausages, jams, marmalade and honey.

Burgers with stir-fried vegetables & red rice

It's easy to make home-made beef or chick-pea burgers. Prepare them while the rice is cooking, then cook the stir-fry. Serves two.

ready in **30** minutes

Beef burgers

200g (7oz) very lean beef mince
1 medium onion, finely chopped
A dash of soy sauce
A large pinch of chilli powder (optional)
1 tablespoon olive oil

Mix the ingredients in a bowl or a mixer. Blend into a paste. Season with freshly ground pepper. Form two 2.5cm (1in) thick burgers. Heat the oil in a pan and cook over a medium heat, turning once.

Stir-fry

300g (10oz) raw vegetables per person, chopped, or 1 packet ready-prepared vegetables

Cook the vegetables in a little water or lemon juice. If you wish, add a sauce after cooking (p.141).

Chick-pea burgers
with a red salsa

Red rice

½ small onion, finely chopped
½ tablespoon olive oil
50g (2oz) red rice
150ml (¼ pint) light vegetable stock

Soften the onion in the oil in a saucepan over a medium heat. Add the rice and stock and simmer for 25 minutes or until the rice is al dente.

Chick-pea burgers

1x400g (13oz) can chick-peas, drained and rinsed
1 small onion, chopped
50g (2oz) carrot, finely grated
2 tablespoons mixed seeds
1 tablespoon olive oil
½ teaspoon ground cumin
A dash of soy sauce

Mash the ingredients with a potato masher in a bowl, or put them in a mixer and blend into a paste. Form into four burgers. Heat the oil in a frying pan and cook over a medium heat until lightly browned on both sides. Serve with a red salsa (p.165).

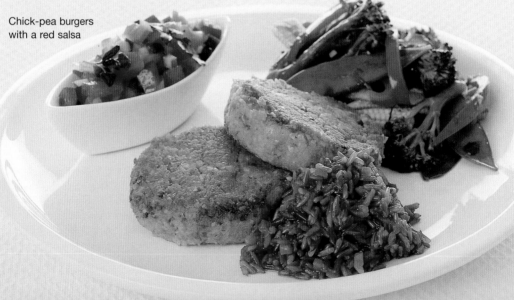

Oat-crumb fish or haloumi, sweet potato & salad

Preparing your own flavoured crumbs is cheap and simple. For this recipe, bake a large sweet potato and make the salad first. Serves two.

ready in 30 minutes

Oat-crumb fish fillets
with half a baked sweet
potato & a green salsa

Oat-crumb fish fillets

200g (7oz) white fish fillet (cod, haddock, etc.)
1 egg, beaten with 1 tablespoon mustard
4 heaped tablespoons oat flakes
1 tablespoon mixed dried herbs (Herbes de Provence)
1 tablespoon olive oil

Ask for the skin to be removed, or lie the fish skin-side down on a chopping board and use a sharp knife, blade horizontal and pointing away from you, to ease the flesh away from the skin.

Lightly beat the egg and mustard. Blitz the oat flakes in a blender for a few seconds to make a coarse powder. Mix it with the dried herbs. Put the egg and oat flakes on two separate flat plates.

Gently heat the oil in a frying pan. Coat the fish in the egg, then the oat flakes. Fry the fish on each side for 3 minutes or so. Serve with lemon wedges, a green salsa (*p.165*), a mixed salad and half the sweet potato each, drizzled with a little olive oil.

Oat-crumb haloumi

1 egg, beaten with 1 tablespoon mustard
4 heaped tablespoons oat flakes
1 tablespoon mixed dried herbs (Herbes de Provence)
1 tablespoon olive oil
200g (7oz) haloumi, cut into 6 slices approx ½cm (¼in) thick (cut the thin end to make long strips)

Lightly beat the egg and mustard. Zap the oat flakes in a blender for a few seconds to make a coarse powder. Mix it with the dried herbs. Put the egg and oat flakes on two separate flat plates.

Gently heat a tablespoon of olive oil in a frying pan. Coat the haloumi slices in the egg mix and then the oat flakes. Fry until the crumbs are brown, when the cheese will be soft and hot. Serve with lemon wedges, a green salsa (*p.165*), a mixed salad and half the sweet potato each, drizzled with a little olive oil.

Soup recipes

Make two soups: two are summer soups (p.34), two winter (p.35). If you wish, make and freeze extra quantities in individual servings to use later in the month. One serving is 250ml (8fl oz).

Light vegetable broth

ready in **20** minutes

100g (3½oz) carrots
100g (3½oz) baby corn
100g (3½oz) baby leeks (or spring onions)
1.2 litres (2 pints) vegetable stock
100g (3½oz) mangetout
2.5cm (1in) cube fresh ginger root, finely grated
1x400g (13oz) can cannellini beans, rinsed and drained
2 tablespoons lemon juice
1 tablespoon dry apple juice
1 teaspoon soy sauce
1 teaspoon miso paste
Tabasco to taste
A small bunch fresh coriander, chopped

Slice the carrots into large matchsticks. Cut the baby corn in half lengthways and across. Cut the leeks or spring onions diagonally in fine slices.

Pour the hot stock into a saucepan, add the carrots and cook for 2 minutes. Add the mangetout and leeks and grated ginger. Simmer together for about 10 minutes. Add the cannellini beans and heat for a couple of minutes. Stir in the lemon juice, apple juice, soy sauce, miso paste, Tabasco and fresh coriander. Once the soup is cool, freeze or refrigerate until needed.

Chilled summer soup

ready in **20** minutes

1 medium red onion, chopped
1 pepper, deseeded and chopped
½ cucumber, chopped
1x400g (13oz) can tomatoes
1 tablespoon lemon juice
1 tablespoon olive oil
1 tablespoon tomato purée
300ml (½ pint) vegetable juice
A good stem of parsley and a couple of sprigs of basil
Finely chopped spring onion, cucumber and tomato to garnish
200g (7oz) quinoa
400ml (¾ pint) light vegetable stock

Put all the ingredients except the quinoa, stock, herbs and vegetable garnish into a blender and blitz until smooth. Stir in the garnish and herbs. Simmer the quinoa in the stock until cooked. Allow to cool, then stir into the soup. Freeze or refrigerate until needed.

Chilled summer soup

Light vegetable broth

Tomato & mixed vegetable soup

ready in **30** minutes

2 tablespoons olive oil
1 medium onion, diced
2 sticks celery, finely sliced
1 fat clove garlic, crushed
1 large red pepper, deseeded and chopped
1x400g (13oz) can plum tomatoes, chopped
½ teaspoon paprika
1 teaspoon mango powder (or juice ½ lemon)
1 litre (1¾ pints) vegetable stock
1x400g (13oz) can cannellini beans, drained and rinsed
A few sprigs of fresh basil, shredded (or 1 teaspoon dried)

Heat the olive oil in a large saucepan. Add the onion, celery, garlic and pepper and cook gently until the vegetables begin to soften. Stir in the tomatoes, paprika and the mango powder (or lemon juice). Simmer for about 5 minutes. Add the stock and cook at a gentle simmer for about 20 minutes until the vegetables are cooked but not soggy. Stir in the cannellini beans and heat for 2–3 minutes. Add in the basil and season with freshly ground black pepper. Once cool, freeze or refrigerate until needed.

Carrot, leek & watercress soup

ready in **30** minutes

1 tablespoon olive oil
1 small onion, chopped
500g (1lb 2oz) carrots, chopped
1 medium leek, finely sliced
1x400g (13oz) can chick-peas, rinsed and drained
1 teaspoon ground cumin
1 litre (1¾ pints) vegetable stock
2 bunches watercress, chopped

Heat the oil in a saucepan and gently soften the onion. Add the carrots and leek and cook for 5 minutes. Add the chick-peas, cumin and stock. Simmer until the carrots are al dente. Tip into a blender, add the watercress and blend until smooth; add more stock if the mix is too thick. Add freshly ground black pepper to taste. Once cool, freeze or refrigerate until needed.

Carrot, leek & watercress soup

Tomato & mixed vegetable soup

Shopping list for storecupboard foods

This list is repeated on page 182 for you to take shopping with you. You may need to replace some of these items during the month.

- [ ] Barley flakes, 1 packet
- [ ] Buckwheat flour, 1 packet
- [ ] Quinoa flakes, 1 packet
- [ ] Quinoa seeds, 1 packet
- [ ] Rice, wholegrain puffed, 1 packet
- [ ] Oatcakes, approx. 4 packets
- [ ] Rye biscuits, approx. 2 packets
- [ ] Corn pasta shells, 1 packet

- [ ] Quinoa, 1 packet
- [ ] Lentils, dried puy, 1 packet
- [ ] Lentils, red, 1 packet
- [ ] Dried sea vegetables (optional) 1–2 packets
- [ ] Dried seaweed, 1 packet
- [ ] Mixed seeds, 1 tub (if not already bought for prep days) OR 1 packet each sunflower, sesame, pumpkin & linseeds to mix (see page 51)
- [ ] Sesame seeds, 1 small packet
- [ ] Sunflower seeds, 1 small packet
- [ ] Cashew nuts, raw unsalted, 1 small packet
- [ ] Mixed nuts, raw unsalted, 1 packet

- [ ] Herb teas, 1–2 packets (peppermint, rooibosch, lemon and camomile are best)
- [ ] Apricots, dried, 1 packet
- [ ] Raisins, 1 small packet
- [ ] Balsamic vinegar, 1 bottle
- [ ] Cider vinegar, 1 bottle

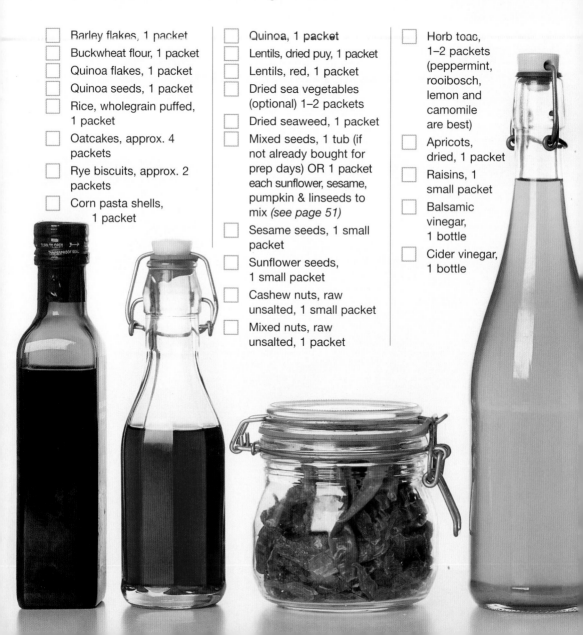

- [ ] Olive oil, 1 bottle (if not already bought for prep days and soups)
- [ ] Sesame oil, 1 bottle
- [ ] Soy sauce, 1 bottle (if not already bought for prep days and soups)
- [ ] *Butter beans, 1x400g (13oz) can
- [ ] *Cannellini beans, 1x400g (13oz) can
- [ ] *Chick-peas, approx. 5x400g (13oz) cans
- [ ] Coconut milk, 1x400g (13oz) can (or 50g/2oz creamed coconut)
- [ ] *Lentils, 1x400g (13oz) can
- [ ] *Mixed beans, 1x400g (13oz) can
- [ ] Passata, 1x500ml (17fl oz) carton

- [ ] *Puy lentils, 1x400g (13oz) can
- [ ] Plum tomatoes, approx. 2x400g (13oz) cans
- [ ] *Red kidney beans, 1x400g (13oz) can
- [ ] Black olives, 1 jar
- [ ] Dijon mustard, 1 pot
- [ ] Five-spice paste, 1 jar (also called Chinese five-spice paste)
- [ ] Five-spice powder, 1 jar (also called Chinese five-spice powder)
- [ ] Hot horseradish
- [ ] Mixed roast peppers, 1 jar
- [ ] Sun-dried tomatoes, 1 jar
- [ ] Tamarind paste, 1 jar
- [ ] Tabasco sauce (or cayenne pepper), 1 bottle
- [ ] Tapenade, 1 jar
- [ ] Thai fish sauce, 1 bottle
- [ ] Worcestershire sauce, 1 bottle

- [ ] Black peppercorns, 1 packet
- [ ] Black mustard seeds, 1 packet
- [ ] Caraway (or fennel) seeds, 1 packet
- [ ] Cardamom pods, 1 jar
- [ ] Cayenne pepper, 1 jar
- [ ] Celery seeds, 1 packet
- [ ] Cinnamon powder, 1 jar
- [ ] Cinnamon stick, 1
- [ ] Curry powder, 1 jar
- [ ] Dried dill, 1 jar
- [ ] Mixed dried herbs, 1 jar
- [ ] Nutmeg (fresh or dried)
- [ ] Turmeric powder, 1 jar
- [ ] Yeast-free bouillon powder, 1 tub (if not already bought for soups and prep days)

*All cans should be free from added salt and sugar

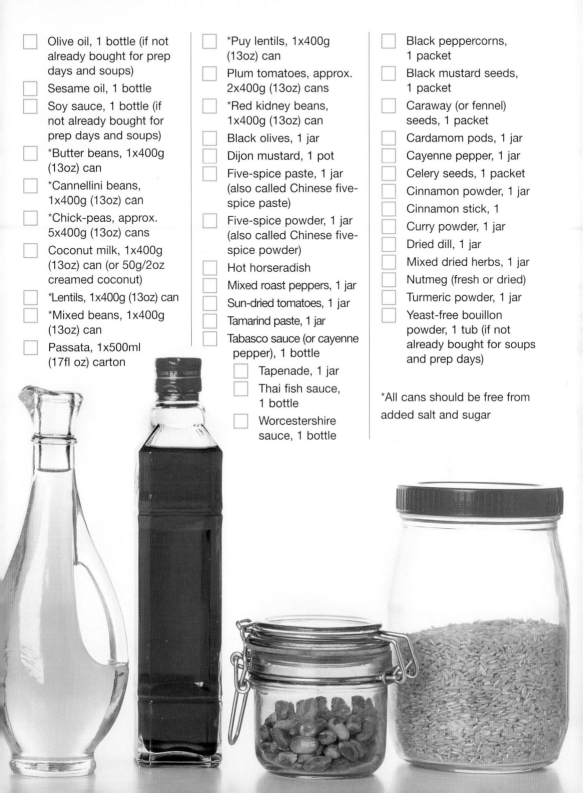

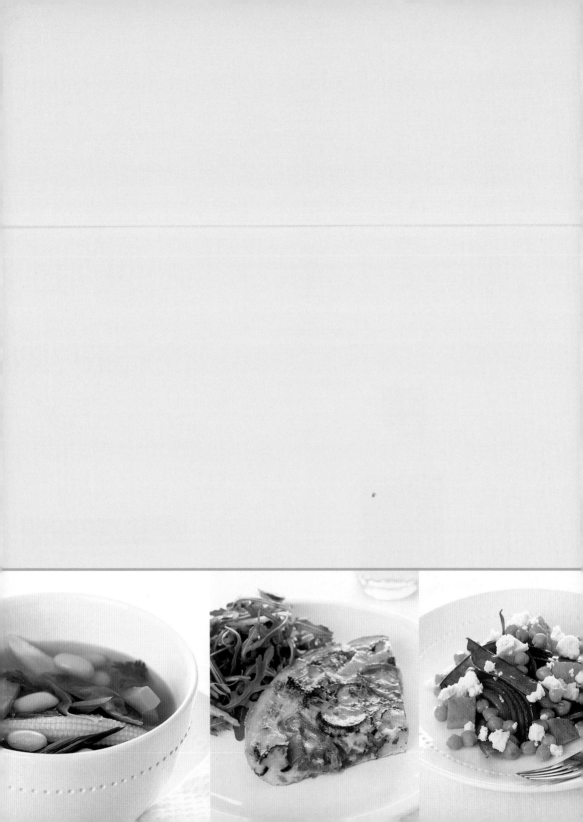

Week 1: fresh start

This first week is a new seven-day plan that incorporates my 10 Principles *(pp.136–37)* and is designed to kick-start your new approach to eating. It's not the easiest week, but it can work wonders for even the most hardened dieters.

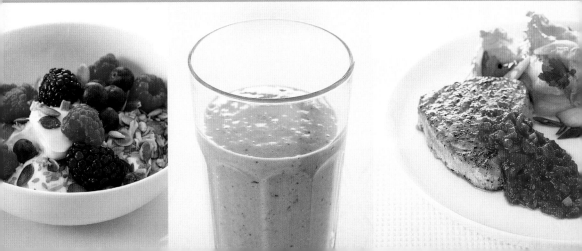

Fresh start: Ian's advice

For some of you, this coming week may be a complete departure from how you usually eat, in which case you may find the plan a little harder; for others, this week may be relatively easy. It all depends on what you have been eating in the past.

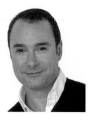

Week 1 is designed to start on a Thursday. During this week you'll be introduced to a healthy, filling diet based on my 10 Principles *(pp.136–37)*. Whilst I don't believe in long-term "hardcore" dieting, these first seven days are slightly restrictive and may prove tough for some of you. However, I have given you a set plan and all the recipes to make it easier to follow.

Be prepared

Preparation is vital on this plan – to guarantee success, you need to be mentally prepared to make changes and ensure that you have the right foods. Shopping lists are provided for this reason. Remember, too, to buy suitable containers to take food and drinks to work.

This week may be a complete **departure** from how you usually eat

The Food Doctor daily routine

Your day starts with a hot lemon and ginger drink to stimulate your digestion and liver function. It also helps educate your palate away from sweet tastes. If you rely on tea or coffee in the mornings, it will also help to change your habits and get you used to no caffeine. Breakfast is essential, but can cause problems if you are used to eating a bowl of sugary cereal in double-quick time. Getting up just ten minutes earlier will make the difference between having time to prepare breakfast and finding this week relatively simple, or struggling through and risking failure.

A word on the juice and smoothie snacks: my recipes provide nutrients and flavour, and home-made is always preferable. If you can't make a juice or smoothie every day, I've given you a couple of easy substitutes – but don't make these a regular fixture.

I've tried to keep lunches simple, using reserved portions of food from your evening meals or defrosted soups from the batches you've made during your preparation days. I've also included time-saving tips for making dinners, but do look ahead and check the ingredients and methods a day or so beforehand. This is when preparation is so important to your success on this plan.

I hope you enjoy this week. If you find it difficult, bear in mind that you are on the first step of a plan that will bring you many benefits, not to mention weight loss. You can also read the experiences of the Diet Club members for encouragement and moral support.

Shopping list for week 1, days 3–9

This shopping list includes approximate quantities for all meals and snacks in Week 1.

This list is repeated at the back of the book for your convenience: just rip out page 183 to take shopping with you.

- [ ] Apples, approx. 7
- [ ] Berries, fresh or frozen, approx 600g (1lb 3½oz)
- [ ] Lemons, 12
- [ ] Oranges, 6
- [ ] Pears, approx. 7
- [ ] Pomegranate, 1 (optional)
- [ ] Asparagus spears, 12 (or 2 plump heads of red or green chicory)
- [ ] Butternut or acorn squash, 1 (or choose any other firm-fleshed squash)
- [ ] Carrots, small, 1
- [ ] Courgettes, medium, 1
- [ ] Garlic, 1 bulb
- [ ] Mangetout, 150g (5oz)
- [ ] Mixed raw vegetables, approx. 500g (1lb) or equivalent weight of ready-prepared vegetables in packets
- [ ] Mixed salad ingredients: enough for 6 portions
- [ ] Onions, small, 3
- [ ] Pepper (yellow or green), 1
- [ ] Red onion, medium, 1
- [ ] Red peppers (Romano if possible), 2
- [ ] Rocket leaves (optional), 1 packet
- [ ] Shallots, 3
- [ ] Spring onions, 1 bunch
- [ ] Sprouted seeds (if not growing your own), 1 tub
- [ ] Tomatoes, medium-large, 3 (or 1 small can chopped tomatoes)
- [ ] Watercress, fresh, 1 bunch
- [ ] Basil, fresh, 1 bunch
- [ ] Coriander, fresh, 1 bunch
- [ ] Fresh root ginger, 1 large-sized piece
- [ ] Parsley, fresh, 1 bunch
- [ ] Sage, fresh, 1 bunch
- [ ] Cottage cheese (optional), 1 large tub
- [ ] Feta cheese, 1 pack
- [ ] Haloumi, 1 packet
- [ ] Hen's eggs, 11
- [ ] Live natural low-fat yoghurt, 1 large pot
- [ ] Milk, whole or semi-skimmed, 1 pint
- [ ] No-fat soft cheese, 1 large tub
- [ ] Parma ham (or good-quality ham), 4 thin slices (if using ham, day 5)
- [ ] Reduced-fat fromage frais, 1 tub
- [ ] Tofu, 200g (7oz) (if making Spicy tofu, day 7)
- [ ] Rye bread, 1 loaf
- [ ] Wholemeal bread, 1 loaf
- [ ] Apple juice, dry or unsweetened, 1 carton
- [ ] Carrot juice, fresh, 725ml (1¼ pints)
- [ ] Mixed vegetable juice, 725ml (1¼ pints)
- [ ] Nut or soya milk, approx. 550ml (19fl oz)
- [ ] Chicken joints (leg and thigh), 2 (if making Spicy chicken, day 7)
- [ ] Tuna steaks, 2, approx. 100g (3½oz) each (if making Tuna in spicy tomato sauce, day 4)
- [ ] Plum tomatoes, 1x200g (7oz) can (if making Tuna in spicy tomato sauce, day 4)
- [ ] Light vegetable stock, 1.2 litres (2 pints)

week 1
day 3

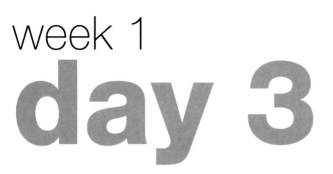

Breakfast

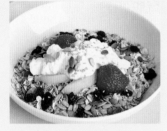

Hot lemon & ginger drink

1 slice ginger (or ½ cinnamon stick)
Juice ½ lemon
Boiling water to fill a tumbler

Put the ginger or cinnamon and juice in the tumbler. Add water. Leave until cool enough to drink.

Toasted cereal with yoghurt, seeds & fruit

30g (1oz) toasted cereal *(p.51)*
3 tablespoons live natural low-fat yoghurt
1 tablespoon mixed seeds (pumpkin and sunflower)
2 tablespoons seasonal fruit, such as berries, or 1 apple, chopped

Combine the ingredients in a bowl. Add some milk, or milk substitute, to make the mix a little thinner to suit your taste.

Morning snack

250ml (8fl oz) Vitamin juice

1 rye cracker spread with no-fat soft cheese

To make the Vitamin juice, see page 65. Add fresh watercress if you are using a vitamin juice mix that you prepared previously.

To make no-fat soft cheese more interesting, try the flavourings suggested below. If you want to substitute no-fat soft cheese with something else, try low-fat fromage frais, cottage cheese or feta cheese.

Flavoured no-fat soft cheese spreads

1 tablespoon no-fat soft cheese
¼ teaspoon hot horseradish, or a sprinkle of ground cumin, or ½ teaspoon (to taste) of tapenade
A squeeze of lemon juice

Mix either the horseradish, cumin or tapenade with the cheese and add a little lemon juice to taste.

Lunch

Carrot, leek & watercress soup, or Light vegetable broth, with 1 slice of rye bread

All soup recipes are listed on pages 34–35. If you haven't made up a batch of soup in advance, do so now and freeze the remaining portions until needed.

"I love the fact that I am not having to spend extra money buying lunches"
Rachael

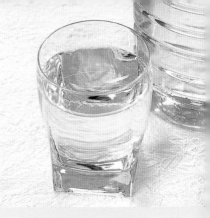

The Food Doctor

Tip for the day ...

If you are off to work, prepare your snacks, drinks and lunch at breakfast time to take with you in plastic containers or flasks.

Afternoon snack

250ml (8fl oz) Fruit smoothie

1 tablespoon mixed seeds, such as sesame, sunflower and pumpkin seeds *(or see p.51)*

To make the Fruit smoothie, see page 65. Either add the seeds to the smoothie mix as you blitz it in a blender, or eat them separately.

Dinner

Roast vegetables with chick-peas *(p.58)*

Save a portion for lunch on day 5

This recipe uses acorn squash, which is usually available for most of the year, but any firm-fleshed squash in season is also suitable.

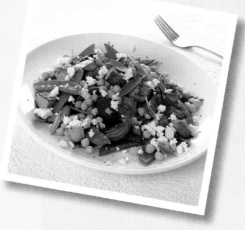

Stay hydrated

Keeping your fluid intake consistently high is vital if you want to lose weight. Water is the best and the most effective way of staying hydrated through the day. You should aim to drink at least 1.5 litres (3½ pints) or more of water a day – that's about six generously sized glasses (or eight normal glasses). You should increase this amount during hot weather or when you are exercising.

There's little difference between choosing tap, bottled mineral or filtered water, but be aware that the gas contained in sparkling bottled mineral water can encourage bloating and discomfort in the gut. Stay hydrated is Principle 2 of The 10 Food Doctor principles *(pp.136–37).*

week 1
day 4

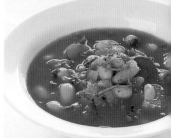

Breakfast

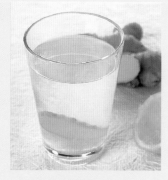

Hot lemon & ginger drink *(p.42)*

Apple porridge with yoghurt & sunflower seeds

50g (2oz) toasted oat flakes
150ml (¼ pint) water
25ml (1fl oz) dry apple juice
2 tablespoons live natural low-fat yoghurt
1 teaspoon sunflower seeds
A pinch cinnamon powder

Gently simmer the oat flakes with the water and apple juice. Serve with the yoghurt, sunflower seeds and a pinch of cinnamon to taste.

Morning snack

250ml (8fl oz) Vitamin juice

1 apple with a small piece of feta cheese

To make the Vitamin juice, see page 65. Add fresh watercress if you are using a vitamin juice mix that you prepared previously.

The size of feta cheese you have should be a small square – about 3x3cm (1¼x1¼in), which is approximately 40g (1¼oz) – but you don't need to weigh it. Just use your judgement and enjoy eating your snack.

"The snacks between meals are keeping me full, so I don't crave chocolate or other sweet treats" Katie

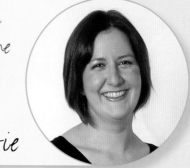

Lunch

Tomato & mixed vegetable soup, or Chilled summer soup, with 1 slice of rye bread

The recipes for all the soups are listed on pages 34–35.

The Food Doctor

Tip for the day ...

If you've chosen to eat lentils tonight, you could cook double the quantity and store half of it in the fridge for dinner on day 6.

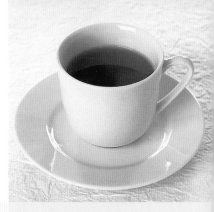

Afternoon snack

250ml (8fl oz) Fruit smoothie

1 tablespoon mixed seeds, such as sesame, sunflower and pumpkin seeds *(or see p.51)*

To make the Fruit smoothie, see page 65. Either add the seeds to the smoothie mix as you blitz it in a blender, or eat them separately.

Dinner

Tuna or lentils in spicy tomato sauce *(p.59)*

Fresh tuna is an excellent source of essential fatty acids and protein, while cooked tomatoes are high in health-giving properties.

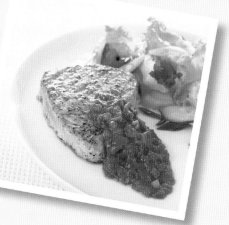

What to drink

Herb teas such as peppermint tea are an excellent choice of drink in addition to drinking plain water. These drinks can count towards your total daily fluid intake. Most fruit teas taste quite sweet, so check the ingredients and avoid any brands with added sugar. Good choices of herb or fruit teas include:

☐ Camomile tea
☐ Lemon tea
☐ Peppermint tea
☐ Rooibosch tea

Juices diluted with water and Food Doctor soups can also count towards your daily intake of fluids. While you are following The Food Doctor 30-day diet plan, you should avoid all caffeinated tea and coffee, alcohol and soft fizzy drinks. During week 1 you should also avoid any decaffeinated drinks.

week 1
day 5

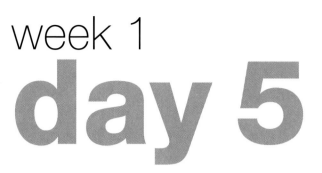

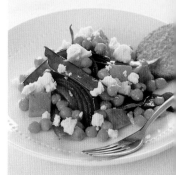

Breakfast

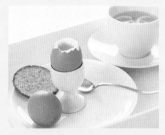

Hot lemon & ginger drink (p.42)

Two boiled eggs with oatcakes

2 medium eggs
1 or 2 oatcakes, spread sparingly with butter if you wish

Bring a small saucepan of water to the boil and place the eggs in the pan, one at a time, using a tablespoon. Boil your eggs according to your personal preference; the ideal time to cook a soft-boiled egg is four minutes. Serve the eggs and oatcakes with your morning cup of hot lemon and ginger.

Morning snack

250ml (8fl oz) Vitamin juice (p.65)

1 oatcake generously spread with houmous (below)

Home-made houmous

1x400g (13oz) can chick-peas, rinsed and drained
2 cloves garlic
3 tablespoons lemon juice
3 tablespoons olive oil
2 tablespoons sesame oil
2 teaspoons soy sauce

Put the ingredients in a food processor. Blitz until smooth. Season with freshly ground black pepper. Add more soy sauce, or lemon juice to taste. For an interesting texture, stir in 1 tablespoon of toasted sesame seeds. Cover and store in the fridge for up to five days.

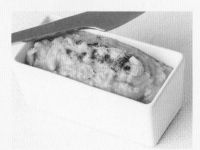

Home-made houmous

Lunch

Roast vegetables with feta cheese

2 tablespoons roast vegetables reserved from dinner, day 3
50g (2oz) feta cheese
1 oatcake

Crumble the feta cheese over the roast vegetables and serve with the oatcake.

> "The Roast vegetables & feta cheese tasted really delicious with some extra sage added"
>
> Lynne

The Food Doctor

Tip for the day ...

If you tend to feel hungry again a couple of hours after eating dinner, save a small portion of your meal to eat as a late snack.

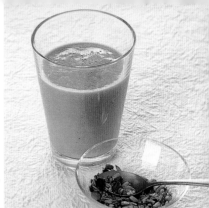

Afternoon snack

250ml (8fl oz) Fruit smoothie

1 tablespoon mixed seeds, such as sesame, sunflower and pumpkin seeds *(or see p.51)*

To make the Fruit smoothie, see page 65. Either add the seeds to the smoothie mix as you blitz it in a blender, or eat them separately.

Dinner

Crumbed asparagus with ham or haloumi & salad *(p.60)*

This recipe uses asparagus in a different way: roasted rather than steamed. Eating asparagus regularly can help maintain healthy bacteria in your digestive system.

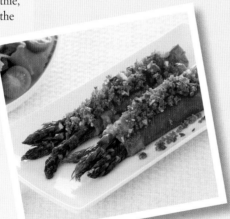

Alternative snacks

If you happen to forget to make your own vitamin juice or smoothie, or end up being on the go all day, try these substitutes – but only occasionally, as buying ready-made produce is not ideal.

For an alternative vitamin juice, buy a can of vegetable juice and have 250ml (8fl oz) with 1 tablespoon of mixed seeds and a couple of sprigs of watercress. If you have a blender to hand, blitz these ingredients together with a squeeze of lemon juice or a slice of fresh ginger.

To make a substitute smoothie, buy a fresh, ready-made fruit smoothie that contains no banana, yoghurt or added sugar. Mix the smoothie with 75ml (3fl oz) nut milk, 2 tablespoons of no-fat soft cheese and a squeeze of lemon. Measure 250ml (8fl oz) and have the smoothie with 1 tablespoon of mixed seeds.

week 1
day 6

Breakfast

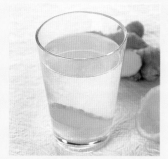

Hot lemon
& ginger drink *(p.42)*

Apple & pear porridge with yoghurt

50g (2oz) oat flakes
150ml (¼ pint) water
25ml (1fl oz) dry apple juice
2 tablespoons live natural low-fat yoghurt
1 pear, cored and chopped

Gently simmer the oat flakes with the water and apple juice. Serve with the yoghurt and chopped pear on top.

Morning snack

250ml (8fl oz) Vitamin juice

1 tablespoon flavoured or plain no-fat soft cheese or houmous with crudités or 1 oatcake

To make the Vitamin juice, see page 65. Add fresh watercress if you are using a vitamin juice mix that you prepared previously.

If you are on the go today and need a more instant snack, have an apple or a pear with six or seven raw, unsalted nuts, such as almonds, walnuts and Brazil nuts.

Lunch

Carrot, leek & watercress soup, or Light vegetable broth, with 1 slice of rye bread

All soup recipes are listed on pages 34–35.

> I've enjoyed the soups for lunch. For extra tang, I added some lemon juice to today's soup"
>
> Mary

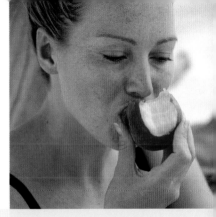

The Food Doctor

Tip for the day ...

To give your meal tomorrow night a stronger flavour, marinate either the tofu or chicken tonight *(see p.62 for ingredients)*.

Afternoon snack

250ml (8fl oz) Fruit smoothie

1 tablespoon mixed seeds, such as sesame, sunflower and pumpkin seeds *(or see p.51)*

To make the Fruit smoothie, see page 65. Either add the seeds to the smoothie mix as you blitz it in a blender, or eat them separately.

Dinner

Warm lentil salad *(p.61)*

Save a portion for lunch tomorrow

Lentils are a valuable source of vegetable protein, minerals and soluble fibre. Puy lentils taste wonderfully rich and meaty, which adds to the big flavours in this dish.

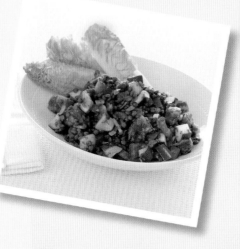

Make time to eat

Eating is obviously essential, but it's also meant to be pleasurable. Many of us lead such busy lives that we treat most of the meals we eat like fast food: we eat as quickly as possible in order to move onto the important tasks of the day.

If you stop what you're doing and make time to eat, the benefits are huge: you reduce your stress levels and gain a feeling of satisfaction that you've eaten a tasty, filling meal. Chew your food slowly and thoroughly so that you digest your food properly and maintain good digestive health. Your body can then absorb the nutrients effectively. Make time to eat is Principle 9 of The 10 Food Doctor principles *(pp.136–37)*.

week 1
day 7

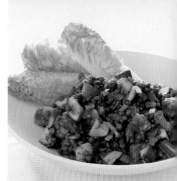

Breakfast

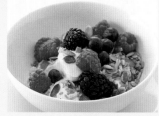

Hot lemon & ginger drink (p.42)

Yoghurt with toasted oat flakes or puffed rice, seeds & fruit

4 tablespoons live natural low-fat yoghurt
1 tablespoon toasted flakes or puffed rice *(see recipe, right)*
3 tablespoons mixed seeds
½ pomegranate or 2 tablespoons of mixed berries if in season

Put the yoghurt into a bowl and add the toasted cereal and seeds. Loosen the pomegranate seeds by gently squeezing the fruit and easing out the red seeds with a fork, avoiding the yellow pith. Spoon the pomegranate seeds or berries over the top and serve.

Morning snack

250ml (8fl oz) Vitamin juice

1 rye biscuit generously spread with flavoured or plain no-fat soft cheese (p.42), houmous (p.46) or cottage cheese

To make the Vitamin juice, see page 65. Add fresh watercress if you are using a vitamin juice mix that you prepared previously.

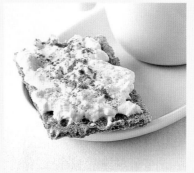

Cottage cheese on rye biscuit

Lunch

Lentil salad

1 portion Lentil salad reserved from dinner, day 6
Your choice of salad dressing (pp.143,145,147)
A small side salad (optional)

Drizzle a little of the salad dressing over the lentil salad, add a few lettuce leaves if you wish and serve.

"The Lentil salad is one of the nicest things I've eaten in ages"
Brendan

The Food Doctor

Tip for the day ...

To prolong the shelf life of your batches of toasted cereals and seeds, store the airtight jars in a cool, dark place.

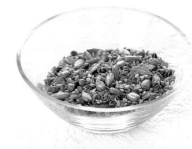

Afternoon snack

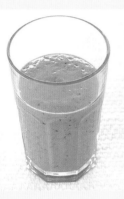

250ml (8fl oz) Fruit smoothie

1 tablespoon mixed seeds, such as sesame, sunflower and pumpkin seeds *(or see p.51)*

To make the Fruit smoothie, see page 65. Either add the seeds to the smoothie mix as you blitz it in a blender, or eat them separately.

Dinner

Spicy tofu or chicken with steamed rainbow vegetables *(p.62)*

Choose a colourful mix of seasonal vegetables for this meal. Brightly coloured fruit and vegetables provide high levels of beneficial nutrients, while soya and chicken are both ideal sources of lean protein.

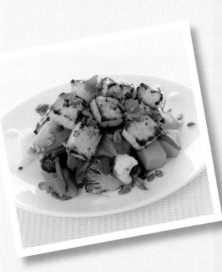

Preparing a batch

Toasted flakes or rice

125–250g (4–8oz) oat flakes or wholegrain puffed rice, depending on how big a batch you want to make

Preheat the oven to 180°C/350°F/gas mark 4. Spread the flakes or rice on a baking sheet. Cook for 20 minutes, turning occasionally. Once browned, leave to cool and store in an airtight jar.

Toasted cereal & Toasted seeds

For the cereal:
50g (2oz) quinoa seeds
50g (2oz) quinoa flakes
100g (3½oz) barley flakes
100g (3½oz) oat flakes
50g (2oz) raisins

For the seeds:
1 tablespoon each quinoa seeds, sesame seeds, pumpkin seeds, sunflower seeds, poppy seeds

Heat a heavy, dry pan until hot. Toast each seed or cereal for a few minutes until browned. Toss regularly. Leave to cool. When the cereal is cool, stir in the raisins. Store in airtight jars.

week 1
day 8

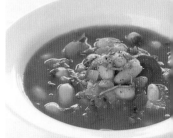

Breakfast

Hot lemon & ginger drink *(p.42)*

Spicy mixed flake porridge

1 star anise

100ml (3½fl oz) boiling water

30g (1oz) mixed flakes (use a mix of large and small flakes: oats, millet, quinoa, barley, rice, etc)

¼ teaspoon ground cinnamon

Juice ¼ lemon

1 tablespoon live natural low-fat yoghurt

1 apple, cored and grated

Rind ¼ orange

Sunflower seeds (optional)

Put the star anise into a jug and pour in the boiling water. Leave to stand for 5 minutes. Put the flakes in a pan, add the ground spice, lemon juice and water and stir well. Simmer gently for 3 minutes, or until the flakes are soft and the mix is a thick but soft consistency. Stir in the yoghurt. Serve topped with the apple, orange rind and seeds.

Morning snack

250ml (8fl oz) Vitamin juice

1 oatcake generously spread with houmous *(p.46),* flavoured or plain no-fat soft cheese or cottage cheese

To make the Vitamin juice, see page 65. Add fresh watercress if you are using a vitamin juice mix that you prepared previously. If you don't have time to make your own houmous, try to buy organic houmous. The quality of olive oil used in organic products is usually better, which gives you some beneficial essential fats.

Lunch

Tomato & mixed vegetable soup, or Chilled summer soup, with 1 slice of rye bread

The recipes for both soups are listed on pages 34–35.

"I'm amazed I don't want to eat anything else; I've had no desire to go to the snack machine at work"

Karen

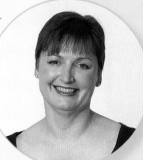

Tip for the day ...

Don't use lack of time as a reason not to exercise. Factor some activity into your day for the best possible results.

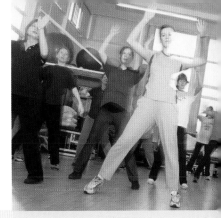

Afternoon snack

250ml (8fl oz) Fruit smoothie

1 tablespoon mixed seeds, such as sesame, sunflower and pumpkin seeds *(or see p.51)*

To make the Fruit smoothie, see page 65. Either add the seeds to the smoothie mix as you blitz it in a blender, or eat them separately.

Dinner

Frittata & green leaves *(p.63)*

Save a portion for lunch tomorrow if you wish

Egg dishes make a filling and satisfying fast meal, so it's always worth keeping some eggs in the fridge as an essential standby ingredient.

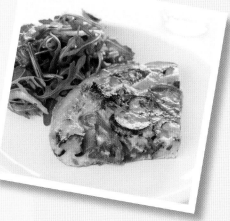

Exercise is essential

It's hard to find time to exercise if your week is busy, but fitting in a brisk walk every day, or a couple of workouts a week at the gym, will mean that your success rate on this diet will be much better than if you do nothing at all.

Any exercise that raises your heart rate consistently for a minimum of 20 minutes is ideal. And while exercise is essential, movement is even more crucial: take the stairs at work or walk to the next bus stop to keep physically active. But don't overdo things: if you over-exercise, your metabolic rate may actually slow down in time.

Have a small snack before and after you exercise to sustain your energy levels *(see also p.134)*. Exercise is essential is Principle 7 of The 10 Food Doctor principles *(pp.136–37)*.

week 1
day 9

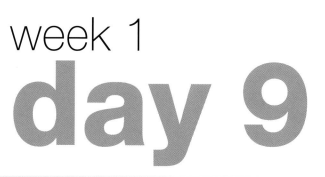
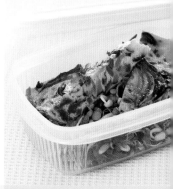

Breakfast

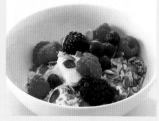

Hot lemon & ginger drink *(p.42)*

Your choice of cereal breakfast

Cereal recipes are listed on pages 42, 44, 48, 50 and 52.

Morning snack

250ml (8fl oz) Vitamin juice

1 apple with a small piece of feta cheese

To make the Vitamin juice, see page 65. Add fresh watercress if you use a juice mix you prepared previously. If you have to make a substitute juice, see page 47.

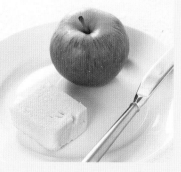

Lunch

Frittata or Chick-pea salad

1 portion reserved Frittata from dinner, day 8 with 2 tablespoons sprouted seeds, a dressing *(pp.143,145,147)* and 1 slice bread, OR

1 tablespoon canned chick-peas, 4 cherry tomatoes, 2 tablespoons sprouted seeds and a dressing, 1 tablespoon mixed seeds *(p.51)* and 1 slice bread

Drizzle the dressing over the frittata or salad and serve with the bread on the side.

"The frittata tasted really good – I used leftovers from the fridge so there was no waste"

Rachael

Tip for the day ...

You can buy ready-grown sprouted seeds in the shops, but if you want to grow your own sprouted seeds, see page 151.

Afternoon snack

250ml (8fl oz) Fruit smoothie

1 tablespoon mixed seeds, such as sesame, sunflower and pumpkin seeds *(or see p.51)*

To make the Fruit smoothie, see page 65. Either add the seeds to the smoothie mix as you blitz it in a blender, or eat them separately.

Dinner

Egg-fried quinoa

Either save a portion of egg-fried quinoa or reserve some raw vegetables for lunch tomorrow

If you'd prefer not to include egg in tonight's recipe, marinate 150g (5oz) tofu in soy sauce and lemon juice, cook it under the grill and add it to the dish.

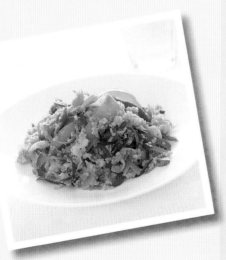

Health check

This is the end of your first full week on the diet. You may be experiencing headaches, mild diarrhoea, spots or lethargy, but these symptoms should soon pass. If you have water retention, try drinking dandelion tea.

On the other hand, you may already be experiencing some positive benefits:

- ☐ Reduced cravings for caffeine, sugar and/or alcohol
- ☐ Improved digestion
- ☐ Enhanced absorption of ingredients
- ☐ More energy
- ☐ Improved sense of well-being

Don't worry if some or all of these beneficial effects don't apply to you yet – it's different for everyone.

Week 1 diary

During week 1, keep track of the foods and recipes that you're enjoying, and how you are feeling. Tick off each day as you go, and make a daily record of how you're coping and whothor you aro becoming aware of any major or minor changes to your health.

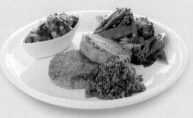

	DAY 3
☐	What I've enjoyed eating/How do I feel?

- -

- -

- -

- -

- -

- -

- -

- -

- -

- -

DAY 6

☐ What I've enjoyed eating/How do I feel?

DAY 7

☐ What I've enjoyed eating/How do I feel?

DAY 4

What I've enjoyed eating/How do I feel?

DAY 5

What I've enjoyed eating/How do I feel?

DAY 8

What I've enjoyed eating/How do I feel?

DAY 9

What I've enjoyed eating/How do I feel?

Roast vegetables & chick-peas with feta cheese | DINNER DAY 3

This meal is deliciously crunchy and filling. Butternut squash is a good alternative if you can't find acorn squash. Try using a vegetable peeler to take off the skin.
Serves two.

250g (8oz) red onion
250g (8oz) acorn (or other firm-fleshed) squash
1–2 tablespoons olive oil
2–3 sprigs fresh sage (or ½ teaspoon dried sage)
150g (5oz) mangetout, rinsed
1x400g (13oz) can chick-peas, rinsed and drained
(reserve 1 tablespoon for day 8 dinner)
100g (3½oz) feta cheese, crumbled

Heat the oven to 180°C/350°F/gas mark 4. Peel and slice the red onion coarsely from top to bottom. Peel and cut the squash into cubes.

Heat a tablespoon of olive oil in a roasting tin, add the onions and toss well. Cook for 10 minutes. Add the squash and the sage, mix well and cook for a further 15 minutes. Add the mangetout and chick-peas, mix well and add another tablespoon of olive oil if necessary. Cook for a further 5 minutes.

Remove 2 heaped tablespoons of the roast vegetables to save for lunch on Day 5. Divide the remainder onto two plates, top with the crumbled feta and a little chopped sage and serve.

Tuna or lentils in spicy tomato sauce

The tomato sauce for this dish is very spicy. If you prefer a milder sauce, reduce the quantity of chilli powder you use or leave it out altogether. Serves two.

ready in 30 minutes

1 tablespoon olive oil, plus extra for brushing tuna
2 shallots, peeled and chopped
½ teaspoon smoked paprika
¼ teaspoon chilli powder (or to taste depending on the strength of the powder)
1x200g (7oz) can chopped tomatoes
1 teaspoon tomato purée
1 clove garlic, crushed
Juice ½ orange
1 teaspoon balsamic vinegar
2 tuna steaks (approx. 100g/3½oz each) or 150g (5oz) puy lentils and 400ml (¾ pint) light vegetable stock (if you make the stock too strong, the lentils taste salty)

To cook the tuna:

Cook the tomato sauce first, then brush each steak with a tablespoon of olive oil and cover with a good grinding of fresh black pepper. Wrap each steak tightly in foil. Heat a heavy-based pan until very hot. Put the wrapped tuna in the pan and press down hard to cook it. Turn over and repeat. Cook for approximately 5 minutes on each side. Unwrap and serve with the sauce and a large green salad.

To cook the lentils:

Cook the lentils first, then the sauce. Simmer the lentils in the stock in a medium-sized saucepan, uncovered, for about 25 minutes, or until all the fluid has been absorbed. Stir the tomato sauce into the lentils and serve with a large green salad.

To make the spicy tomato sauce:

Heat a tablespoon of olive oil in a small saucepan over a medium heat. Add the shallots and let them soften for a few minutes. Turn the heat down a little if they brown too quickly. Add the paprika and chilli powder and stir quickly. Add the tomatoes, tomato purée and garlic, stir well and bring the sauce to simmering point. Stir in the orange juice and vinegar and simmer gently for 5 minutes to allow the flavours to blend well.

Tuna in spicy tomato sauce

Crumbed asparagus with ham or haloumi & salad

DINNER DAY 5

If asparagus is not in season, try baking two heads of chicory until tender in a shallow dish half-filled with vegetable stock. Serves two.

ready in 25 minutes

12 spears fresh asparagus, tough ends snapped off
1–2 teaspoons olive oil
4 thin slices of Parma ham (or a good-quality cooked ham) or 4 thin slices haloumi

For the topping:
1 clove garlic, chopped or crushed
1 thick slice rye bread
1 teaspoon mixed toasted seeds *(p.51)*
Grated zest ½ orange
1 teaspoon olive oil

Preheat the oven to 200°C/400°F/gas mark 6. Wash the asparagus spears thoroughly, put them in a baking tray, add a teaspoon or so of olive oil and lightly coat each spear in the oil. Roast for 10–12 minutes until just tender.

While the asparagus cooks, make the topping: either blitz all the ingredients in a small chopper, or grate the breadcrumbs, crush the seeds in a pestle and mortar and add the other ingredients.

Group the roasted spears in four bundles of three spears each. If using ham, wrap each bundle in one slice of ham. Top each parcel with some crumb mixture and brown gently under the grill for 5 minutes or so. Serve with a mixed salad.

If using haloumi, cover each bundle with one slice of haloumi. Top each parcel with some crumb mixture and brown gently under the grill for about 5 minutes. Serve with a mixed salad.

Crumbed asparagus with ham

Warm lentil salad

DINNER DAY 6

If time is short in the evening, you can use a can of lentils, and chop the pepper, onion and courgette in advance. Reserve a portion for lunch tomorrow. Serves two.

150g (5oz) dried puy lentils (or 1x400g/13oz can puy lentils)

400ml (¾ pint) very light vegetable stock (if cooking dried puy lentils) with 1 thick slice lemon added

1 tablespoon olive oil

1 small onion, chopped

1 clove garlic, peeled

1 medium courgette, cubed

1 red pepper (such as Romano), chopped

3 good-sized, ripe tomatoes, skinned and chopped (or in winter use 1x200g/7oz can chopped tomatoes)

1 teaspoon balsamic vinegar

2.5cm (1in) fresh ginger, grated (optional)

A small bunch fresh basil or coriander, chopped

1 tablespoon mixed seeds *(p.51)*

Simmer the dried lentils in the stock and lemon for 25–30 minutes until the stock is absorbed. Top up with water if the stock boils away too fast. Discard the lemon slice.

Heat the oil in a frying pan or wok. Gently soften the onion, then add the garlic, courgette and pepper. Stir over a medium heat for a few minutes until they begin to soften, but still have a bite. Add the tomatoes, vinegar and ginger, and season with freshly ground black pepper. Cook until all the vegetables are piping hot.

Combine with the lentils, stir in the fresh herbs, add a spoonful of seeds and serve with a fresh green salad on the side.

If you would prefer to have this with extra protein, serve it with some grilled haloumi or Tapenade fish fillets *(p.174)*.

Spicy chicken or tofu with rainbow vegetables

If you can marinate the tofu or chicken overnight, the flavours will be more intense. Otherwise, marinate the ingredients for a minimum of 15 minutes. Serves two.

ready in **30** minutes

2 chicken joints (leg and thigh), skinned, with the flesh scored a couple of times, or 200g (7oz) tofu, cut into cubes
3–4 good sprigs fresh coriander, chopped
A few mixed seeds

For the marinade:
½ onion or 2 large shallots
2 cloves garlic, peeled
2.5cm (1in) fresh ginger, peeled and chopped
½ teaspoon ground cumin powder
Juice and grated zest ½ lemon
4 tablespoons live natural low-fat yoghurt

For the vegetables:
300g (10oz) mix of vegetables per person, cut into small chunks or 1 packet ready-prepared vegetables

Blitz the onion or shallot, garlic, ginger and cumin in a blender (or grate the onion and ginger and crush the garlic). Add the lemon and yoghurt and stir. Season with freshly ground black pepper Add the tofu or rub the marinade into the chicken joints and leave to marinate.

If using chicken, preheat the oven to 180°C/350°F/gas mark 4. Place the chicken into a baking dish, cover with foil and cook for about 30 minutes until the juices run clear, but the chicken isn't dried out.

Put the vegetables in a steamer and steam for 10–15 minutes until they are just cooked, but not soft.

If using tofu, set the grill at medium hot and grill the pieces of tofu for a few minutes on each side until golden brown.

Divide the vegetables between two plates and pile on the chicken or tofu. Heat the remaining marinade, drizzle over each plate and serve with chopped coriander and seeds scattered on top.

Spicy tofu with rainbow vegetables

Frittata & green leaves

Buy a jar each of sun-dried tomatoes and peppers and use some frozen peas if you don't have time to roast vegetables tonight. Save a portion for lunch tomorrow. Serves two.

ready in **30** minutes

250g (8oz) mix of vegetables, chopped
1 tablespoon olive oil, plus a little extra to cook the onion
1 small onion, sliced
6 medium hen's eggs
1 tablespoon live natural low-fat yoghurt
1 tablespoon canned chick-peas, rinsed and drained
A handful fresh parsley or coriander, chopped

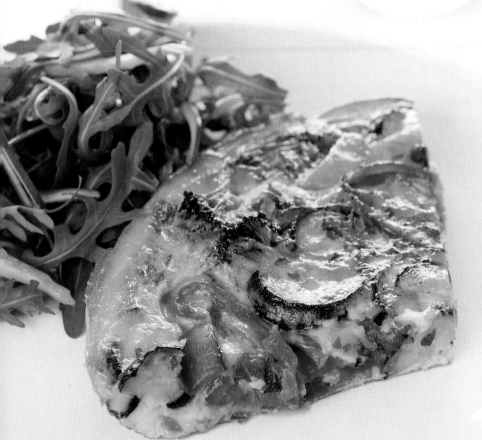

Preheat the oven to 180°C/350°/gas mark 4. Use a small roasting tin to toss the mixed vegetables in a tablespoon of olive oil and roast for about 20 minutes until cooked. Cook the onion in a large omelette pan in a little olive oil until soft. Whisk the eggs and yoghurt, add the chick-peas and pour onto the onions. Stir in the roasted vegetables. Season with freshly ground black pepper, add chopped parsley or coriander and stir. Allow to cook gently until the bottom is set, then slip the pan under a medium grill to brown the top. Serve with a salad of green leaves.

Egg-fried quinoa

DINNER DAY 9

The quinoa can be cooked in advance and stored in the fridge if you need to save time cooking tonight. Serves two.

ready in **30** minutes

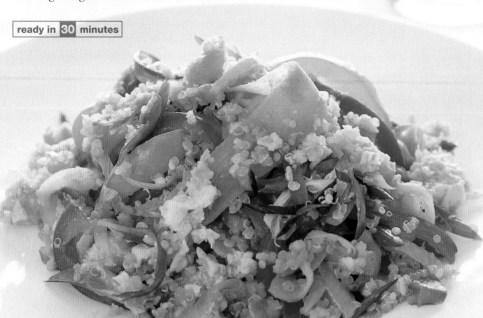

150g (5oz) quinoa
300ml (½ pint) very light stock
1 clove garlic, peeled
3 medium hen's eggs
2 tablespoons olive oil, plus a little to cook the eggs
1 large shallot
2 cloves garlic
½ or ¼ teaspoon chilli powder (to your own taste)
1 small onion, finely sliced
1 tablespoon lemon juice
1 small carrot, sliced into ribbons using a potato peeler
1 red pepper, deseeded and finely sliced
1 yellow or green pepper, deseeded and finely sliced
3 spring onions, shredded
1 tablespoon soy sauce

Simmer the quinoa in the stock with the garlic clove for about 20 minutes, until it is cooked and the fluid is absorbed. Then mash in the garlic.

Scramble the eggs, using a little oil, in a non-stick pan or wok until firm.

Blend the shallot, garlic and chilli powder in a blender (or grate the shallot and crush the garlic).

Heat a tablespoon of olive oil in a wok and cook this paste over a gentle heat for a few minutes. Add more oil and the onion, and cook for 5 minutes or so. Add the lemon juice, carrot and pepper and cook for a couple of minutes until they soften. Stir in the spring onions, soy sauce, quinoa and egg, cook until piping hot and serve.

Snacks

The quantities for each recipe should make one serving, 250ml (8fl oz), but you can double the quantities to make enough for two days.

Fruit smoothie

ready in **2** minutes

80g (3oz) berries (either fresh or frozen)
1 apple or 1 pear, peeled and cored (or ½ each)
2 tablespoons no-fat soft cheese
75ml (3fl oz) nut or soy milk
A squeeze of lemon juice
A pinch of cinnamon

Put all the ingredients into a blender and blitz until smooth. If the mix is too thick, add a little water. The cinnamon gives the smoothie a good flavour and helps to balance blood sugar levels.

Vitamin juice

ready in **2** minutes

100ml (3½fl oz) mixed vegetable juice
100ml (3½fl oz) carrot juice
4–5 good sprigs fresh watercress
Juice ½ orange
Juice ½ lemon

Put all the ingredients into a blender and blitz until the watercress is finely chopped. If you make the mix in advance, leave out the watercress and add it fresh each day.

To add flavour, try these ingredients alone or in combination, in any proportion, to suit your taste: grated ginger (good for digestion), fennel or caraway seeds (good for digestion), celery seeds (good for blood cleansing), ground cinnamon (good for insulin function), cayenne (good for digestion).

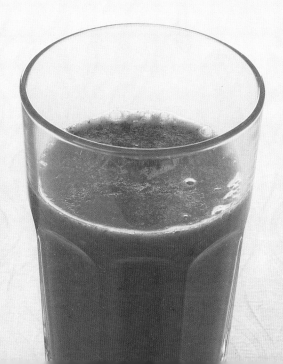

Diet Club diaries

Keeping a diary while you're on The Food Doctor Diet plan enables you to assess each day, analyze how you're feeling and note down which foods you're enjoying. Here our Diet Club members record their experiences of week 1.

Mary says "The snacks have really helped me. The only time I've felt hungry is later at night, but that's because I had got into a regular habit of grazing all evening. My routine was sabotaged on day 5 when I had to take the car in early to the garage for emergency repairs. I only had my hot lemon drink before I left, but there was nothing to eat or drink at the garage. By lunchtime I was feeling headachy and craving chocolate and carbohydrates. I found it hard to get back on track the rest of the day."

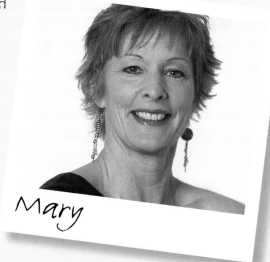

Mary

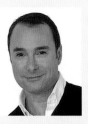

Ian says "This first week is all about changing your eating habits and embarking on a new and positive approach to the way you view your relationship with food. Week 1 can be tough going for some people because it's such a big change from their previous eating routine – as Mary has found in the evenings as she begins to kick her old habits. Aside from the evenings, I am pleased that Mary hasn't felt hungry and, if anything, this fact has served to highlight how much she was previously eating out of habit, not hunger. Experiencing feelings of fatigue a couple of days into The Food Doctor Diet plan is quite normal, although eating snacks has really helped keep Mary's glucose levels stable (which is also a large part of avoiding hunger) so she hasn't mentioned feeling fatigued. Mary was thrown off course on day 5 by not having food with her, so her glucose levels were low. Of course, it's quite normal to feel dizzy and headachy if you haven't eaten, but it's interesting to note how Mary immediately wanted chocolate to compensate. This really goes to show how important it is to eat little and often, and, if at all possible, to have a snack with you at all times – even if it's just an apple and a bag of unsalted nuts. You could keep them in the glove compartment of the car, or in your bag or briefcase, and remember to re-stock should you have occasion to use up your store."

Brendan says "This week has gone better than I thought. The food is tasty, I'm not hungry, and I'm more awake and sleeping better. One major thing I'm not enjoying is dull headaches; on some days they've been quite severe."

Ian says "Brendan has taken to this plan really well, and although the headaches are not uncommon, they should pass quite quickly. Sleeping well and awakening feeling refreshed makes a significant difference to overall energy levels and my method of combining the food groups is working well for him."

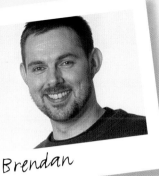

Brendan

Joan says "It's been a tough week with all that shopping and preparation, but I've enjoyed the recipes so far and they are much tastier than I thought. The biggest change for me is waking up and staying awake instead of falling asleep again in the mornings; I was up and about at 8.30am on Sunday!"

Ian says "The first week isn't easy, especially if, like Joan, you have got out of the habit of making food for yourself. I am pleased that Joan is enjoying the food, and even more so that she finds it tasty. It's great to see that Joan feels so awake in the mornings; her days are so much longer now!"

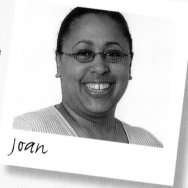

Joan

Jon says "I had quite a bad headache, but it's lessening now. I didn't realize how much time is spent preparing "proper" food, but it was fun cooking the meals and I enjoyed eating them. I'm finding it hard to remember to chew my food thoroughly, as I'm sure I just used to swallow my food whole."

Ian says "Headaches in week 1 are common, but, like the other Diet Club members, Jon's headaches are now on the way out. As Jon says, preparing food can take time, but it's enjoyable too. This time spent really is a worthwhile investment."

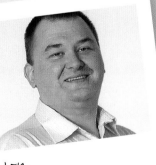

Jon

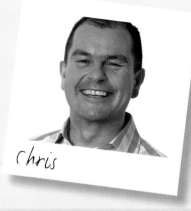

Chris

Chris says "One of the concerns I had about the plan was going without caffeine, but I'm not missing it. Since starting week 1, I've had no acid stomach and I feel great. The secret of cooking the recipes seems to be in preparing all the ingredients up front. And the meals taste delicious."

Ian says "When you start a plan, it's easy to focus on what you can't have, assuming that you'll miss it. Chris was probably using caffeine to get a quick boost of energy; now that his glucose levels are maintained with regular snacks and meals, he simply has less need for it."

Karen says " I have found the food lovely and I haven't been tempted to eat anything else, which is amazing! My family is enjoying the meals too, so I haven't had to cook two different meals. I'm feeling lethargic and bloated with water retention, but my PMS symptoms are much improved."

Ian says "It's unusual to experience water retention and bloating, but anything is possible in the first week. The symptoms will quickly pass though. Finding that the food is satisfying does seem to be a revelation to Karen, as her previous food intake was far from ideal before. It's also great to note that she isn't having cravings for the types of food she used to eat."

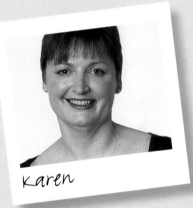

Karen

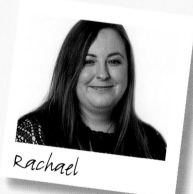

Rachael

Rachael says "I'm not missing anything about the foods I used to eat and I'm not hungry at all. I'm really in the swing of getting everything ready before it's needed so there's no rushing about. I think being organized is key to this lifestyle."

Ian says "Rachael is doing so well. She has grasped the principles and her experience demonstrates that preparation is key. Whilst not always possible, if you can get some preparation done beforehand (even if it's as simple as preparing vegetables) you'll have the greatest success and the easiest time."

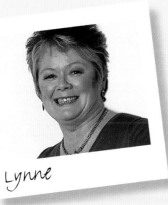

Lynne

Lynne says "I feel fit and well, I'm sleeping great and I've had no indigestion at all. I had bad headaches at the start, but now I just feel a bit emotional and tetchy. The first week was a challenge, but I have a pressure cooker so the soups were made in five minutes."

Ian says "I am pleased that Lynne hasn't had any indigestion, and I'm confident that the headaches and bad mood will pass quickly. These symptoms can affect many people; to reduce the chance of it happening to you, ensure that you never miss a meal or snack."

Katie says "Following the recipes has helped me to eat correct portion sizes and to stop eating when I'm full, rather than finishing my plate. People at work have already noticed my face has more of a glow than usual. It's probably because I'm drinking about 2 litres of water a day."

Ian says "Katie has been following the plan closely, and it's paying off. Drinking plenty of water will encourage healthy-looking skin, and the lack of refined sugars and saturated fats in the new foods she's eating are a contributing factor to that. She already has a sense of well-being."

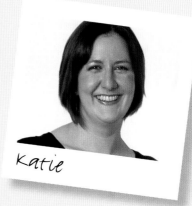

Katie

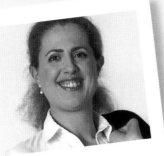

silvia

Silvia says "One week on and I have to say I feel well. The first days without my morning coffee and chocolate bars were hard, and I had a constant headache and itchy spots. Now they have gone. I've been quite disorganized and tired as I have a young daughter so I'm simplifying the meals."

Ian says "Silvia is adapting the meals to suit her lifestyle, which is a good move so long as she is still enjoying the food and the ratios between carbohydrates and protein are unaltered. As you can see, food cravings do pass, so stick with it."

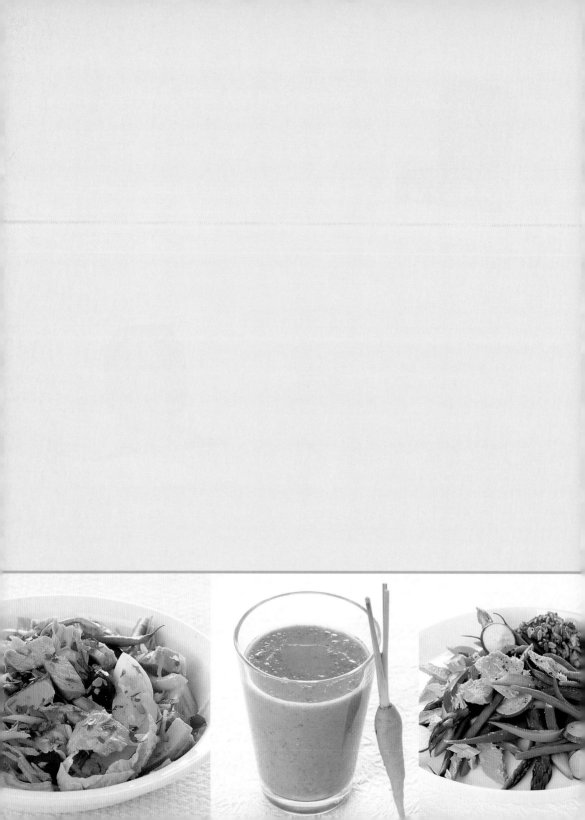

Weeks 2 & 3: readjusting

The following two weeks show how adaptable my plan is, as there are more choices for meals and snacks. Any side-effects experienced in the first week should now be a thing of the past, and you will really begin to see my principles in action.

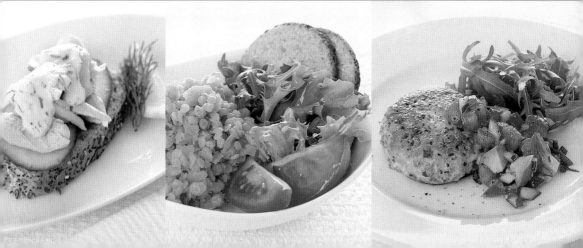

Readjusting: Ian's advice

Congratulations on getting through the first week. If you found week 1 challenging, you'll be pleased to hear that weeks 2 and 3 are more easy going, allowing you a little more freedom in what you can eat.

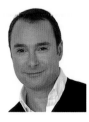

A good diet has innumerable benefits, so investing some time and thought into what you eat has to be a worthwhile exercise. If you found the first week especially tough then I am delighted you have got this far. The harder you found it, the more it suggests that your diet really needed some attention. The discipline that the first week demands is a useful exercise in understanding the level of priority that food has been for you in the past. Many clients report that after the first couple of days of being on my Food Doctor Diet plan, they find they get into the habit of preparing and planning food a little way in advance. They are often shocked to realize how little time they had previously spent on organizing and eating their food.

Dealing with choice

The good news is that things get easier from here on. You will be able to mix and match to suit your tastes, something that I know was popular with some of The Food Doctor Diet Club members in this book. If you flick through the next few pages, you will see that I'd still like you to start the day with the hot lemon and ginger drink, but that the breakfasts are more varied. You'll also be continuing with the mid-morning and mid-afternoon snacks, although it's up to you to choose what you want to eat from the selection of juice, smoothie and snack recipes that I've provided.

One or two Diet Club members found that the prescriptive nature of the first week suited them really well, and they were somewhat daunted by the choice that this next stage affords. If you find yourself feeling a little anxious about what's in store over the next two weeks, my advice is simple. Now that you have some flexibility in your routine, it's worthwhile reminding yourself often that you should be asking, "Where's my protein?" every time you make a decision about what to eat. If

Ask yourself, "**Where's my protein**?" every time you **decide** what to **eat**

you keep this simple mantra in mind, you will find it much easier to stay within the guidelines of the plan and reap the benefits.

All in all, this gradual process of readjusting to a better way of eating should enable you to become accustomed to the extra effort of choosing the right types of food for yourself. There has been some really encouraging feedback from the Diet Club members of their experiences in weeks 2 and 3, with comments ranging from "shopping for food is now more fun and stimulating", to "my awareness of foods around me is improving". Overall, there

There's been a **growing** sense of **confidence** when making **food** decisions

has been a sense of growing confidence from them when it comes to making great food decisions and planning ahead for meals.

Coping with difficult situations

For those of you who do shift work, I can appreciate that ensuring that you eat every two and a half to three hours can be a problem. I suggest that, without fail, you take care to plan ahead. Bear in mind that half an apple and a palmful of mixed seeds or nuts will do as a snack, and they are foods that can easily be slipped into your pocket or bag. This may not make for an exciting snack, but as we all have to adapt the food we can eat around our work and family commitments, this is probably the best solution.

I also know that weekend afternoons can be a problem when you have less to occupy yourself with than usual. You might want to think back to what you had for brunch or lunch and check that it was correctly balanced with the right food types to ensure a slow and consistent level of blood glucose. If you truly are hungry, you may need to tweak your lunchtime accordingly or, if you had brunch,

I suggest that you have a small extra snack, such as sliced fruit with some sort of protein. If you find that you are eating or wanting to eat out of boredom, then please find something to do. It's an easy answer, but distracting yourself may really be the best way.

If you have kids and are tempted to eat their tea, I recommend that you cook them food that you can also eat as a snack without veering away from the plan.

Late evenings can be a problem too, and in many ways this highlights the fact that in the past you may have been eating out of boredom rather than hunger. If you are hungry, then a little leftover dinner as a small snack should suffice, even if it's just a couple of mouthfuls. Some Diet Club members found that making themselves a cup of herbal tea satisfied their need to get something from the kitchen, so consider that option too.

It's been of great interest to me to have so many Diet Club members following my plan at the same time. I am more accustomed to working on a one-to-one basis with clients, and I'm there to support them should they require it. The Diet Club members formed their own group and stayed in touch by email, sharing their thoughts and experiences. You may wish to do the same with a group of friends or colleagues, if possible, as it's a great means of moral support for everyone involved.

Sharing **thoughts** and **experiences** is a **great** means of moral **support**

Shopping list for weeks 2 & 3, days 10–23

This shopping list includes approximate quantities for all the supper recipes and weekday lunches. It does not include ingredients for your choice of breakfasts, snacks, or weekend brunches or lunches.

This list is repeated at the end of the book for your convenience: just rip out pages 184–85 to take shopping with you.

FRESH FOOD FOR WEEK 2, DAYS 10–16

- [ ] Lemons, 2
- [ ] Limes, 1
- [ ] Oranges, 2
- [ ] Asparagus, 100g (3½oz)
- [ ] Avocado, 1
- [ ] Beetroot, raw or ready-cooked, 150g (5oz)
- [ ] Carrots, medium, 2
- [ ] Cherry tomatoes, 1 large tub
- [ ] Chicory, medium, 2 (or gem lettuce)
- [ ] Courgettes, medium, 1
- [ ] Fennel, medium, 1
- [ ] Mixed green vegetables, approx. 600g (1lb 3½oz)
- [ ] Mixed raw vegetables (eg, French beans, runner beans, mangetout, asparagus) approx. 450g (15oz)

- [ ] Mixed salad ingredients: enough for 9 portions
- [ ] Mushrooms, small, 150g (5oz), plus 8 mushrooms (if making Vegetable brochettes, day 12)
- [ ] Onions, small, 4
- [ ] Onions, medium, 2
- [ ] Peppers, red, 3
- [ ] Peppers, yellow, 2
- [ ] Root ginger, fresh, 1 large piece
- [ ] Spinach (fresh or frozen) or kale, 100g (3½oz)
- [ ] Sprouted seeds (if not growing your own), 1 tub
- [ ] Coriander, fresh, 1 bunch
- [ ] Parsley, fresh, 1 bunch
- [ ] Feta cheese, 150g (5oz)
- [ ] Haloumi, 200g (7oz) (if making Grilled haloumi, day 10)
- [ ] Hen's eggs, 3
- [ ] Reduced-fat fromage frais, 1 tub
- [ ] Tofu, 200–250g (7–8oz) (if making Smoked tofu salad, day 14)
- [ ] Dry apple juice, 1 carton
- [ ] Chicken thigh fillets, 250–300g (8–11oz) (if making Chicken brochettes, day 12)
- [ ] Duck breasts, 2, approx. 200g (7oz) each (if making Duck breast salad, day 14)

- [ ] Trout, 2, approx. 200g (7oz) after removing the head and tail (if making Baked trout, day 10)
- [ ] Tuna, 1 small can for lunch, day 10, and 1 large can (if you have run out) for lunch day 16

DAY 13 DINNER OPTIONS

Quick country soup

- [ ] Lemons, 1
- [ ] Mushrooms, button, 400g (13oz)
- [ ] Onions, medium, 1
- [ ] Dried sea vegetables, 1 small packet, or spinach, 50g (2oz)
- [ ] Vegetable stock, 500ml (17fl oz)

Four bean salad

- [ ] Lemons, 1
- [ ] Broad beans, 100g (3½oz)
- [ ] Green beans, 100g (3½oz)
- [ ] Mangetout or petit pois, 100g (3½oz)
- [ ] Pepper, 1 (red or orange)
- [ ] Spring onions, 1 bunch
- [ ] Fresh herbs of your choice, 1 bunch
- [ ] Feta cheese, 50g (optional)
- [ ] *Cannellini beans, 1x400g (13oz) can (if you have run out)

FRESH FOOD FOR WEEK 3, DAYS 17–23

- [ ] Lemons, approx. 4
- [ ] Limes, 2
- [ ] Aubergines, 1 (approx. 200g/7oz)
- [ ] Beefsteak tomatoes, 2
- [ ] Carrots, small, 1 (if making Vegetarian burgers, day 23)
- [ ] Cherry tomatoes, 1 tub
- [ ] Courgettes, 500g (1lb)
- [ ] Mixed raw vegetables, approx. 250g (8oz) or equivalent weight of ready-prepared vegetables in packets
- [ ] Mixed salad ingredients: enough for 9 portions
- [ ] Mushrooms, large, 4
- [ ] Onions, medium, 1
- [ ] Shiitake mushrooms, 4 (if making Vegetarian burgers, day 23)
- [ ] Spring onions, 1 bunch)
- [ ] Sprouted seeds, 1 tub (if you are not growing your own)
- [ ] Sweet potatoes, medium, 1
- [ ] Tomatoes, large, 5
- [ ] Coriander, fresh, 1 packet
- [ ] Parsley, fresh, 1 bunch
- [ ] Root ginger, fresh, 1 large piece (if you have run out)
- [ ] Cottage cheese, 1 tub

- [ ] Feta or haloumi cheese, 200g (7oz) (if using cheese, day 22)
- [ ] Hen's eggs, 4 (3 if making Egg noodles, day 21, 1 if making Vegetarian burgers, day 23)
- [ ] Live natural low-fat yoghurt, 1 large pot (if you have run out)
- [ ] Black olives, 8–10
- [ ] Smoked tofu, 100g (3½oz) if making Stir-fry tofu, day 19
- [ ] Tofu, 200g (7oz) (if making Vegetarian burgers, day 23)
- [ ] Rye bread, 1 loaf
- [ ] Chicken, 100g (3½oz) (if making Stir-fry chicken, day 19)
- [ ] Chicken or turkey, minced, 300g (10oz) (if making Chicken burgers, day 23)
- [ ] Salmon fillet, 150–200g (5–7oz) (if making Salmon cakes, day 21)
- [ ] White fish fillet, 250–300g (8–10oz) (if using fish, day 22)

DAY 20 DINNER OPTIONS
Salade niçoise
- [ ] Carrot, medium, 1
- [ ] Gem lettuce or similar, 1
- [ ] Green or runner beans, 100g (3½oz)

- [ ] Pepper, yellow, 1
- [ ] Spring onions, 1 bunch
- [ ] Tomatoes, medium, 2
- [ ] Fresh herbs of your choice, 1 bunch
- [ ] Hen's eggs 1 (2 if making vegetarian option)
- [ ] Black olives, 6–8
- [ ] Tuna steak, fresh, 1 or 1 large can of tuna in spring water (if making traditional Salad niçoise)
- [ ] *Chick-peas, 1x400g (13oz) can (if you have run out and are making Spicy chick-peas)

Leek & potato soup
- [ ] Leeks, large, 1
- [ ] Onions, medium, 1
- [ ] Sweet potato, medium, 1
- [ ] Dried sea vegetables, 1 small packet
- [ ] Quinoa, 100g (3½oz) (if you have run out)
- [ ] Light vegetable stock 250ml (8fl oz)

*All cans should be free from added salt and sugar

week 2
day 10

Breakfast

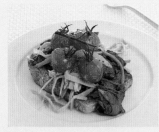

Hot lemon & ginger drink *(p.42)*

Cereal or ham breakfast *(below)*

Cereal recipes are listed on pages 42, 44, 48, 50 and 52.

Sliced ham with tomatoes & spinach

4 cherry tomatoes
A drizzle of olive oil
45g (1½oz) baby spinach leaves
1 thin slice ham, cut into fine strips
1 slice rye or wholemeal toast

Preheat the oven to 180°C/350°F/gas mark 4. Put the tomatoes on a baking tray, and drizzle over a little olive oil. Roast for 10–15 minutes. Meanwhile, steam the spinach. Place the tomatoes, spinach and ham on the toast and serve.

Morning snack

Choose either:

250ml (8fl oz) Vitamin juice (if you have any portions left over from week 1) and 1 oatcake with your choice of spread *(below)*

OR

2 oatcakes or rye biscuits with your choice of spread:

☐ Bean & mustard mash *(p.99)*
☐ Home-made houmous *(p.46)*
☐ Reduced-fat fromage frais & peppers *(below)*
☐ Spicy chick-pea spread *(p.99)*

Reduced-fat fromage frais & peppers

2 tablespoons low-fat fromage frais
2 peppers from a jar, chopped
A squeeze of lemon juice

Spread the fromage frais on two oatcakes. Top with the peppers and a little lemon juice. Store any leftovers in the fridge for up to two days.

Lunch

Egg-fried quinoa

OR

Tuna or tofu salad with seeds

1 portion egg-fried rice reserved from dinner, day 9
OR
1 portion chopped raw vegetables reserved from dinner, day 9
1 tablespoon chick-peas, drained and rinsed
1 small can tuna, drained, or 150g (5oz) smoked tofu
A little dressing *(pp.143,145,147)*

If you are having egg-fried quinoa, serve it cold with a few mixed seeds scattered over the top if you wish. If you are having the tuna or tofu salad, mix all the ingredients together with the dressing and serve.

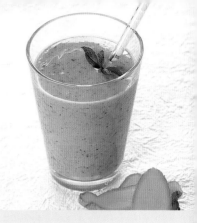

The Food Doctor

Tip for the day ...

Look back to days 3, 4, 6, 7 and 9 for different cereal-based recipes if you don't want ham for breakfast this morning.

Afternoon snack

Choose either:

250ml (8fl oz) High-energy smoothie *(right)*

OR

2 oatcakes or rye biscuits with your choice of spread:

☐ Bean & mustard mash *(p.99)*

☐ Home-made houmous *(p.46)*

☐ Reduced-fat fromage frais & peppers *(see recipe, left)*

☐ Spicy chick-pea spread *(p.99)*

Dinner

Baked trout or grilled haloumi *(p.92)*

Save a portion for lunch tomorrow

Serve your choice of baked trout or haloumi with stir-fried vegetables. If using haloumi, cook the stir fry first.

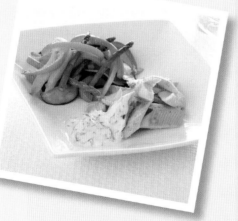

Afternoon snack recipe

All the smoothies listed in week 2 and beyond are complete foods and are good on their own for afternoon snacks. The quantities listed should make 500ml (17fl oz) – enough for two smoothies. If not, top up with a little apple juice. Always store the second portion in the fridge.

High-energy smoothie

½ avocado, stoned and peeled
A small handful fresh watercress
5cm (2in) fresh ginger, grated
2 or 3 sprigs of mint
100ml (3½ oz) water
100ml (3½ oz) dry apple juice
Juice ½ lemon
150ml (¼ pint) live natural low-fat yoghurt

Blend all the vegetables, herbs, water and juices together. Stir in the yoghurt. Do not sieve the smoothie mix as this will remove valuable fibre. If you wish, serve the smoothie with an extra sprig of fresh mint as a garnish.

week 2
day 11

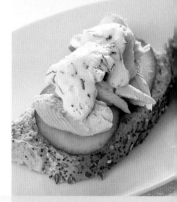

Breakfast

Hot lemon & ginger drink *(p.42)*

Scrambled eggs with toast or oatcakes & sesame seeds

1 teaspoon sesame seeds
2 medium hen's eggs
A dash semi-skimmed milk
A very small knob of butter
1 slice toasted rye or wholemeal bread, or 1 or 2 oatcakes, spread sparingly with butter
A sprig fresh parsley, chopped

Toast the sesame seeds in a small, dry pan over a medium-high heat. Toss the seeds frequently to develop an even colour. Whisk the eggs and milk. Melt the butter in a small pan over a medium heat and cook the eggs. Scatter the seeds and parsley on top of the eggs and serve with the toast or oatcakes.

Morning snack

Choose either:

250ml (8fl oz) Kick-start superjuice *(see recipe, right)*, and 1 oatcake spread with your choice of topping *(below)*

OR

2 oatcakes or rye biscuits spread with your choice of topping:

☐ Bean & mustard mash *(p.99)*
☐ Reduced-fat fromage frais & peppers *(p.76)*
☐ Red lentil & turmeric spread *(p.125)*
☐ Spicy chick-pea spread *(p.99)*
☐ Sweet potato & goat's cheese topping *(p.125)*

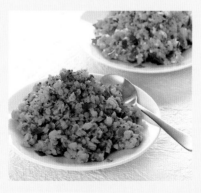

Red lentil & turmeric mash

Lunch

Cold trout or haloumi & your choice of carbohydrate

1 portion cold trout or haloumi reserved from dinner, day 10
1 portion mixed salad or steamed vegetables
Your choice of carbs: 1 slice of rye or wholemeal bread or 2 oatcakes, rice cakes or rye biscuits, or 1 tablespoon rice or quinoa (leftover from a dinner)
A couple of tablespoons of reserved dill sauce or olive oil
A wedge of fresh lemon

Flake the cold trout or cube the haloumi and arrange on a plate with a salad or steamed vegetables and your choice of carbohydrate. Drizzle a little olive oil over the haloumi or the dill sauce over the trout, add a wedge of fresh lemon and serve.

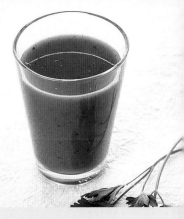

The Food Doctor

Tip for the day ...

If you are making Fruit compote (brunch) and Chicken brochettes (dinner) tomorrow, marinate the ingredients overnight tonight.

Afternoon snack

Choose either:

250ml (8fl oz) High-energy smoothie (if you have portion 2 leftover from yesterday)

OR

2 oatcakes or rye biscuits spread with your choice of topping:

☐ Bean & mustard mash *(p.99)*

☐ Reduced-fat fromage frais & peppers *(p.76)*

☐ Red lentil & turmeric spread *(p.125)*

☐ Spicy chick-pea spread *(p.99)*

☐ Sweet potato & goat's cheese topping *(p.125)*

Dinner

Beetroot risotto with feta cheese & green salad *(p.93)*

Save a portion for lunch tomorrow

Cook the rice and the beetroot at the same time for speed – or alternatively you can use ready-cooked beetroot.

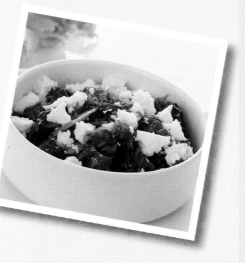

Morning snack recipe

With its mildly spicy undertones of cayenne and paprika, this energy drink is especially good if you are in need of a boost mid-way through the morning. The quantities listed here should make enough for two snacks; if not, top up with tomato juice.

Kick-start superjuice

150ml (¼ pint) carrot juice
100ml (3½fl oz) tomato juice (or ready-mixed vegetable juice)
1 tablespoon lemon juice
A small handful fresh parsley
½ teaspoon cayenne powder
½ teaspoon paprika powder

Put all the ingredients in a food processor and blitz for a few seconds until mixed.

week 2
day 12

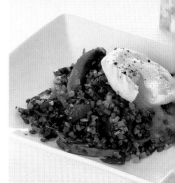

Breakfast

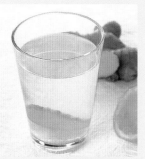

Hot lemon & ginger drink *(p.42)*

If you are having brunch today, eat a small snack at your usual breakfast time.

OR

Your choice of cereal or ham breakfast

Cereal recipes are listed on pages 42, 44, 48, 50 and 52; see page 76 for a ham breakfast recipe.

Morning snack

If you are not having brunch, have the second portion of Kick-start superjuice *(p.79)*, and 1 oatcake spread with a topping:

- ☐ Bean & mustard mash *(p.99)*
- ☐ Classic guacamole *(below)*
- ☐ Reduced-fat fromage frais & peppers *(p.76)*
- ☐ Red lentil & turmeric spread *(p.125)*
- ☐ Spicy chick-pea spread *(p.99)*
- ☐ Sweet potato & goat's cheese topping *(p.125)*

Classic guacamole

2 ripe avocados
2 tablespoons grated onion
1 tablespoon mixed pumpkin, sunflower and sesame seeds
1 small clove garlic, crushed
2 teaspoons lemon juice
2 teaspoons olive oil
A pinch cayenne pepper
A dash of Worcestershire sauce (to taste)
A dash of Tabasco (to taste)

Mash all the ingredients together in a small bowl and season with freshly ground black pepper. Cover tightly with cling film and store in the fridge for up to two days.

Brunch/Lunch

Brunch:
1 livening drink *(right)*, either Fruit compote *(below)* or 1 apple or pear and your choice of brunch *(pp.100–101)*

Fruit compote

6 dried apricots and 5 dried prunes, halved and soaked in 150ml (¼ pint) peppermint tea
50ml (2fl oz) apple juice
½ crisp apple, cored and sliced
½ pear, cored and sliced

Soak the dried fruit overnight. Strain the tea and mix with the apple juice. Combine all the fruits, pour the tea and juice mix over and serve.

OR

Lunch:
Beetroot risotto

1 portion reserved Beetroot risotto from dinner, day 11
Several sprigs watercress
1 hard-boiled egg, quartered
1 slice rye bread

Pile the risotto on top of the watercress, top with the egg and serve with the bread.

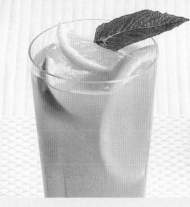

The Food Doctor

Tip for the day ...

You're now allowed a cup of decaffeinated coffee or tea each day if you wish. Ideally, just have one cup, or two cups maximum.

Afternoon snack

Choose either:

250ml (8fl oz) High-energy smoothie *(p.77)* or Fruit smoothie *(p.65)* with 1 tablespoon of mixed seeds

OR

2 oatcakes or rye biscuits with your choice of spread:

☐ Bean & mustard mash *(p.99)*

☐ Classic guacamole *(left)*

☐ Reduced-fat fromage frais & peppers *(p.76)*

☐ Red lentil & turmeric spread *(p.125)*

☐ Spicy chick-pea spread *(p.99)*

☐ Sweet potato & goat's cheese topping *(p.125)*

Dinner

Brochettes *(p.94)*

Include the reserved portion of Beetroot risotto if you had brunch

These brochettes are easy to make and are perfect for cooking either on a barbecue or under the grill.

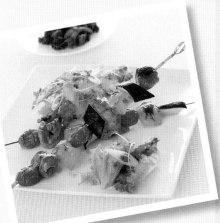

Livening drinks

These fresh tonics are a great way to begin brunch by clearing your palete. Double the quantities to make two servings.

Orange tonic

125ml (4fl oz) freshly squeezed orange juice
125ml (4fl oz) water

Mix the juice and water together and serve chilled.

Fresh juice burst

125ml (4fl oz) chilled carrot juice
125ml (4fl oz) unsweetened or dry apple juice
Juice ½ orange
Juice ½ lemon
A sprig of mint or lemon balm

Mix the ingredients together and serve chilled with the sprig of mint or lemon balm.

week 2
day 13

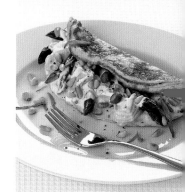

Breakfast

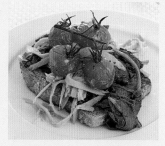

Hot lemon & ginger drink *(p.42)*

If you are having brunch today, eat a small snack at your usual breakfast time.

OR

Your choice of cereal or ham breakfast

Cereal recipes are listed on pages 42, 44, 48, 50 and 52; see page 76 for a ham breakfast recipe.

Morning snack

If you are not having brunch, have 2 oatcakes or rye biscuits with your choice of spread:

- ☐ Bean & mustard mash *(p.99)*
- ☐ Classic guacamole *(p.80)*
- ☐ Home-made houmous *(p.46)*
- ☐ Spicy chick-pea spread *(p.99)*
- ☐ Sweet potato & goat's cheese topping *(p.125)*

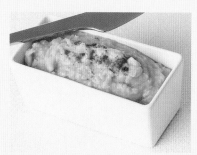

Home-made houmous

Brunch/Lunch

Brunch:
1 livening drink, either Fruit salad *(below)* or 2 apricots and your choice of brunch *(pp.100–101)*

Fruit salad

3 tablespoons fruit salad
2 tablespoons reduced-fat fromage frais
A sprinkling of mixed seeds

Put the fromage frais in a bowl, spoon over the fruit and seeds and serve.

OR

Lunch:
Salmon & steamed vegetables

1 salmon fillet, simply poached or grilled
Approx. 300g (10oz) steamed vegetables
Fresh dill sauce *(p.92)*
Your choice of carbohydrate

Mix up some more sauce if necessary. Serve the salmon with the vegetables, your choice of carbohydrate and the sauce on the side.

The Food Doctor

Tip for the day ...

For a spicy kick, try adding some lemon juice mixed with a teaspoon of olive oil and a few chilli flakes to any dish.

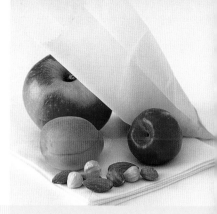

Afternoon snack

Choose either:

250ml (8fl oz) High-energy smoothie *(p.77)* or Fruit smoothie *(p.65)* with 1 tablespoon of mixed seeds

OR

2 oatcakes or rye biscuits with your choice of spread:

☐ Bean & mustard mash *(p.99)*

☐ Classic guacamole *(p.80)*

☐ Home-made houmous *(p.46)*

☐ Spicy chick-pea spread *(p.99)*

☐ Sweet potato & goat's cheese topping *(p.125)*

Dinner

Quick country soup or Four bean salad *(p.95)*

Save two portions of soup for lunch, days 14 and 17, or one portion of salad for lunch, day 14

Freeze the second reserved portion of soup until you need it on day 17.

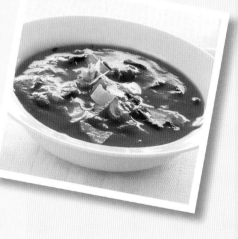

Fuel up frequently

If you have ever felt hungry soon after a meal, you may have found yourself eating more and more. Five small healthy meals, rather than the traditional "three square meals a day", will help you to control what you eat, keep any hunger pangs at bay and maintain your energy levels – hence the all-important fourth Food Doctor Principle, Fuel up frequently.

Ideally, you should eat a light meal every three hours or so. This is why it's important to eat morning and afternoon snacks every day in addition to breakfast, lunch and dinner. Even if you aren't hungry, you really should have something to eat, however small it might be, in order that your metabolic rate is maintained. All The Food Doctor Principles are listed on pages 136–37.

week 2
day 14

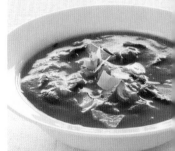

Breakfast

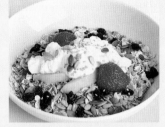

Hot lemon & ginger drink *(p.42)*

Ham or cereal breakfast *(below)*

Other cereal recipes are listed on pages 42, 44, 48, 50 and 52; see page 76 for a ham breakfast recipe.

Millet porridge

30g (1oz) millet flakes
150ml (¼ pint) water
2 tablespoons live natural low-fat yoghurt
1 pear, chopped, but not peeled
1 tablespoon pumpkin seeds

Gently simmer the flakes and water for 5 to 10 minutes until the water is absorbed. Stir in the yoghurt until creamy and serve with the chopped pear and pumpkin seeds on top.

Morning snack

Choose either:

250ml (8fl oz) Kick-start superjuice *(p.79)* and 1 oatcake spread with your choice of topping *(below)*

OR

2 oatcakes or rye biscuits spread with your choice of topping:

- [ ] Bean & mustard mash *(p.99)*
- [ ] Classic guacamole *(p.80)*
- [ ] Home-made houmous *(p.46)*
- [ ] Spicy chick-pea spread *(p.99)*
- [ ] The Food Doctor fresh pesto *(below)*

The Food Doctor fresh pesto

2 tablespoons toasted seeds *(p.51)* or 1 tablespoon each pumpkin and sunflower seeds
3 tablespoons olive oil
A small handful fresh watercress
2 teaspoons lemon juice

Combine the ingredients in a blender and blitz into a thick paste. Add more oil if the paste is too thick. Season with freshly ground black pepper.

Lunch

Soup or salad & your choice of carbohydrate

1 portion Quick country soup or Four bean salad reserved from dinner, day 13
1 tablespoon mixed seeds
1 hard-boiled egg for the salad (optional)
Your choice of carbs: 1 slice of rye or wholemeal bread or 2 oatcakes, rice cakes or rye biscuits, or 1 tablespoon rice or quinoa (leftover from a dinner)

Heat the soup thoroughly and serve with the seeds scattered over the top, or have the remainder of the salad with the egg and mixed seeds. Add your choice of carbs and extra vegetables if you prefer.

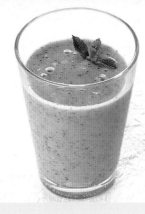

The Food Doctor

Tip for the day ...

If you have any of The Food Doctor fresh pesto left over, it will keep well in the fridge for three or four days for snacks.

Afternoon snack

Choose either:

250ml (8fl oz) Apple & mint smoothie *(right)* or High-energy smoothie *(p.77)*

OR

2 oatcakes or rye biscuits spread with your choice of topping:

☐ Bean & mustard mash *(p.99)*

☐ Classic guacamole *(p.80)*

☐ Home-made houmous *(p.46)*

☐ Spicy chick-pea spread *(p.99)*

☐ The Food Doctor fresh pesto *(see recipe, left)*

Dinner

Duck breast or smoked tofu salad *(p.96)*

Game such as duck is an excellent source of low-fat protein, and is high in iron. If you don't like duck, you can use chicken instead. Tofu is an excellent choice of vegetarian protein.

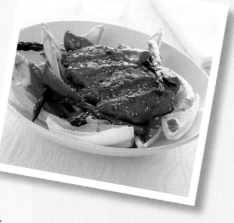

Afternoon snack recipe

This clean-tasting, deliciously refreshing recipe should make 500ml (17fl oz) – enough for two smoothies. If not, top up with apple juice. If you prefer the drink thick, increase the quantities slightly to ensure you have a second smoothie for tomorrow all prepared.

Apple & mint smoothie

1 crisp eating apple, cored and chopped
1 pear, cored and chopped
½ small cucumber
200g (7oz) live natural low-fat yoghurt
A small handful mint leaves
1 tablespoon pumpkin seeds
A squeeze lemon juice

Blend all the fruit, vegetables, herbs, seeds and juice together. Stir in the yoghurt. Do not sieve the smoothie as this will remove valuable fibre.

week 2
day 15

Breakfast

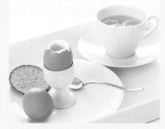

Hot lemon & ginger drink *(p.42)*

Egg or cereal breakfast

Egg recipes are listed on pages 46 and 78; cereal recipes are listed on pages 42, 44, 48, 50, 52 and 84.

Morning snack

Choose either:

250ml (8fl oz) Energizer juice *(see recipe, right)* and 1 oatcake spread with your choice of topping *(below)*

OR

2 oatcakes or rye biscuits spread with your choice of topping:

- [ ] Bean & mustard mash *(p.99)*
- [ ] Classic guacamole *(p.80)*
- [ ] Flavoured no-fat soft cheese spread *(p.42)*
- [ ] Home-made houmous *(p.46)*
- [ ] Spicy chick-pea spread *(p.99)*
- [ ] The Food Doctor fresh pesto *(p.84)*
- [ ] Sweet potato & goat's cheese topping *(p.125)*

Lunch

Mixed sprouted seed salad with avocado & your choice of carbohydrate

3 tablespoons sprouted seeds (p.151)

½ avocado, peeled and cut into chunks

1 tablespoon each of at least two other raw vegetables (whatever you have in the fridge, e.g., peppers, celery, cucumber or cherry tomatoes)

Your choice of carbs: 1 slice of rye or wholemeal bread or 2 oatcakes, rice cakes or rye biscuits, or 1 tablespoon rice or quinoa (leftover from a dinner)

Mix all the ingredients together and serve with your choice of dressing and carbohydrate.

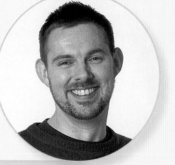

"I had the mixed cereal today. The quinoa seeds give it a great crunchy taste"

Brendan

Tip for the day ...

For an instant snack on the go, buy a pot of houmous and eat with raw vegetable crudités you've prepared at breakfast time.

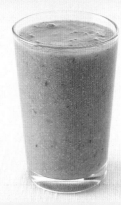

Afternoon snack

Choose either:

250ml (8oz) Apple & mint smoothie (if you have portion 2 leftover from yesterday, day 14) or High-energy smoothie (p.77)

OR

2 oatcakes or rye biscuits spread with your choice of topping:

☐ The Food Doctor fresh pesto (p.84)

☐ Banana & fromage frais spread (below)

Banana & fromage frais spread

½ banana, mashed
1 tablespoon reduced-fat fromage frais
1 teaspoon sesame seeds

Mix the ingredients together and spread on 1 slice of wholemeal or rye bread or 2 oatcakes.

Dinner

Butter beans in tapenade with vegetables (p.97)

Save a portion of steamed vegetables for lunch tomorrow

Like other legumes, butter beans are high in fibre and an excellent source of vegetable protein.

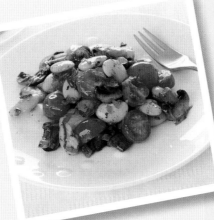

Morning snack recipe

The hint of fresh ginger in this refreshng juice is very beneficial for your digestion. The quantities listed here should make 500ml (17fl oz) – enough for two snacks; if not, top up with carrot or tomato juice. Store the second serving in the fridge until tomorrow afternoon.

Energizer juice

100ml (3½fl oz) carrot juice
100ml (3½fl oz) tomato juice
1 red pepper
Juice 1 orange
Juice 1 lemon
2.5cm (1in) fresh ginger, grated

Put all the ingredients in a food processor and blitz for a few seconds until mixed.

week 2
day 16

Breakfast

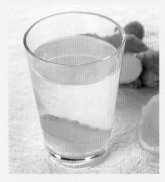

Hot lemon & ginger drink *(p.42)*

Cereal or ham breakfast

Cereal recipes are listed on pages 42, 44, 48, 50, 52 and 84; see page 76 for the ham recipe.

Morning snack

Choose either:

250ml (8oz) Kick-start superjuice *(p.79)* or Energizer juice *(p.87)* and 1 oatcake spread with your choice of topping *(below)*

OR

2 oatcakes or rye biscuits spread with your choice of topping:

- ☐ Bean & mustard mash *(p.99)*
- ☐ Spicy chick-pea spread *(p.99)*
- ☐ Home-made houmous *(p.46)*
- ☐ Reduced-fat fromage frais & peppers *(p.76)*
- ☐ The Food Doctor fresh pesto *(p.84)*
- ☐ Flavoured no-fat soft cheese spread *(p.42)*
- ☐ Egg & crudités *(below)*

Egg & crudités

Approx 100g (3½oz) raw vegetables, such as carrots, peppers, cucumber, cherry tomatoes
1 hard-boiled egg, shelled

Rinse and cut the vegetables into bite-size pieces. Keep the egg and crudités in a sealed plastic container.

Lunch

Tuna & vegetable salad & your choice of carbohydrate

½ large can tuna, drained
1 portion of steamed vegetables reserved from dinner, day 15
Your choice of dressing *(pp.143,145,147)*
Your choice of carbs: 1 slice of rye or wholemeal bread or 2 oatcakes, rice cakes or rye biscuits, or 1 tablespoon rice or quinoa (leftover from a dinner)

Mix the tuna with last night's steamed vegetables. Add some extra raw vegetables if you like and serve with your choice of dressing and carbohydrate.

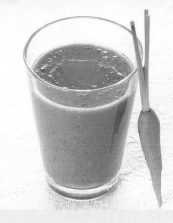

The Food Doctor

Tip for the day ...

The Egg & crudités snack listed here is another great snack if you are on the go: just keep it in your bag until needed.

Afternoon snack

Choose either:

250ml (8oz) Vegetable smoothie *(right)* or Apple & mint smoothie *(p.85)*

OR

2 oatcakes or rye biscuits spread with your choice of topping:

 Cottage cheese

☐ Chick-pea & banana spread *(see recipe, below)*

Chick-pea & banana spread

½ banana, mashed

3 tablespoons chick-peas, drained and rinsed

1 tablespoon reduced-fat fromage frais

A squeeze lemon juice

A pinch cinnamon (optional)

Put the ingredients in a blender and blitz until smooth. Enough for two snacks. Store in the fridge.

Dinner

Carrot & cardamom rice with a green leaf salad *(p.98)*

Save a portion of the rice for lunch tomorrow

An alternative to this recipe, which includes gem squashes, is on page 175.

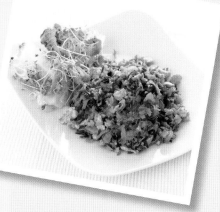

Afternoon snack recipe

If you don't have all the right ingredients for this recipe, try adding whatever is to hand in the fridge such as cooked beetroot, watercress or celery (avoid raw root vegetables though). This recipe should make 500ml (17fl oz) – enough for two smoothies. If not, top up with carrot juice. If you prefer the drink thick, increase the quantities slightly to ensure you have a second smoothie all prepared for tomorrow's snack.

Vegetable smoothie

150g (5oz) cucumber

1 medium tomato

50g (2oz) red pepper

100ml (3½fl oz) carrot juice

Juice 1 lemon

3 tablespoons live natural low-fat yoghurt

Blend the vegetables and juice together for a few seconds in a blender. Stir in the yoghurt. Do not sieve the smoothie as this will remove valuable fibre.

Week 2 diary

If you found week 1 quite tough and restrictive in terms of what you could eat, you should find week 2 easier, as there are more snack options and foods to try. Write down which choices you've made, and any new symptoms or changes you've been noticing.

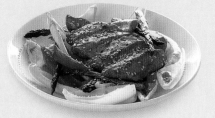

DAY 10
What I've enjoyed eating/How do I feel?

DAY 13
What I've enjoyed eating/How do I feel?

DAY 14
What I've enjoyed eating/How do I feel?

☐ **DAY 11**

What I've enjoyed eating/How do I feel?

- -
- -
- -
- -
- -
- -
- -
- -

☐ **DAY 12**

What I've enjoyed eating/How do I feel?

- -
- -
- -
- -
- -
- -
- -
- -

☐ **DAY 15**

What I've enjoyed eating/How do I feel?

- -
- -
- -
- -
- -
- -
- -
- -

☐ **DAY 16**

What I've enjoyed eating/How do I feel?

- -
- -
- -
- -
- -
- -
- -
- -

Baked trout or haloumi & stir-fried vegetables

DINNER DAY 10

Whether you choose the trout or haloumi option, save a portion for lunch tomorrow. Each recipe serves two.

ready in **30** minutes

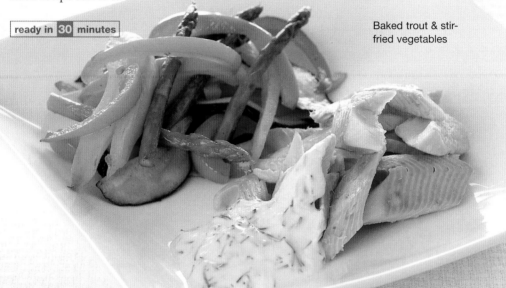

Baked trout & stir-fried vegetables

2 trout, gutted, about 200g (7oz) each with head and tail removed (to allow for cold trout being left over for lunch tomorrow) or 200g (7oz) haloumi, cut into thin slices
1 tablespoon each fresh parsley and coriander

Dill sauce for the trout:
2 tablespoons reduced-fat fromage frais
2 tablespoons horseradish sauce
1 tablespoon lemon juice
1 tablespoon fresh dill, chopped

Heat the oven to 150°C/300°F/gas mark 2. Rinse the fish and fill the cavity with herbs. Wrap each fish loosely in foil and place on a baking tray. Cook for 15–20 minutes until the flesh is opaque, but moist. Cook the stir-fry and mix the sauce. Save a little sauce for lunch tomorrow. Open the parcels, lift the skin from the fish and ease the flesh from the bones. Turn the fish over and repeat on the other side. Serve with the sauce and stir-fry.

For the stir-fry:
300g (10oz) raw vegetables per person, cut into bite-size pieces, or 1 packet ready-prepared vegetables

Optional sauce for the stir-fry:
2cm (¾in) ginger, grated
1 clove garlic, crushed
Grated zest 1 lime
4 tablespoons lime juice
2 tablespoons soy sauce
1 tablespoon balsamic vinegar
1 tablespoon olive oil

Cook the vegetables in a wok over a high heat with a little water or lemon juice until al dente. Add the sauce after cooking.

To make the haloumi:
Once the stir-fry is ready, grill the slices of haloumi until golden. Serve while still hot.

Beetroot risotto with feta cheese & green salad

Supermarkets now sell fresh, ready-cooked beetroot if you want to save time making this dish. You can also cook the rice in advance. Save a portion for lunch tomorrow. Serves two.

500ml (17fl oz) light stock
150g (5oz) rice (red or brown)
1 clove garlic, peeled
1 stick cinnamon
150g (5oz) beetroot, rinsed, or use vinegar-free, ready-cooked beetroot
½ teaspoon caraway seeds, lightly toasted
1–2 tablespoons olive oil
100g (3½oz) spinach or kale, coarsely shredded with thick stems removed
1 medium onion, chopped
1 medium head of fennel, trimmed and cut into medium fine slices
2 teaspoons tamarind paste
150g (5oz) feta cheese, chopped or crumbled

Bring the stock to the boil and add the rice, garlic and cinnamon. Simmer gently, without a lid, for about 35 minutes or until the rice is tender. Drain, remove the cinnamon and mash in the garlic.

While the rice is cooking, cover the beetroot with very lightly salted boiling water and simmer until tender, about 30 minutes. Once cooked, it will be easy to slip off the skins under cold running water and then top and tail the beetroot.

As the rice and beetroot cook, heat a frying pan and lightly toast the caraway seeds. Remove the seeds and add a tablespoon of olive oil to the frying pan. Add the coarsely shredded spinach or kale and cook gently until the leaves have wilted. Remove from the pan and set aside. Add more oil and cook the onion and fennel until golden brown. Stir in the cooked shredded greens, the caraway seeds and tamarind paste. Combine with the rice and beetroot and season with freshly ground black pepper to taste.

Put aside one helping for tomorrow's lunch. Place the remaining risotto in a shallow baking dish and scatter over the feta cheese. Slip into a hot oven for 10 minutes. Serve with a green salad.

Chicken or mixed vegetable brochettes & salad

It's worth marinating the chicken overnight or preparing it in the morning to make the dish tastier. Include the Beetroot risotto if you didn't have it for lunch today. Serves two.

250–300g (8–11oz) chicken thigh fillets, cut into 2 or 3 chunks, or 8 button mushrooms (chestnut mushrooms have a good flavour)
12 baby tomatoes
1 medium courgette, cut into thick slices
1 yellow pepper, cut into chunks

For the marinade:
1 clove garlic, crushed
1 tablespoon dry apple juice
1 tablespoon soy sauce
1 tablespoon tamarind paste
1 tablespoon mustard
A squeeze of lime juice

Mix the marinade. If using chicken, put the chicken pieces and the marinade in a bowl, mix well and leave as long as you can.

Thread the vegetables – and chicken, if you are using it – alternately onto 4 metal or soaked wooden skewers. Brush with olive oil. If you are cooking just vegetables, brush some of the marinade over the prepared skewers. Either cook under a medium grill, or on a barbecue, until the vegetables are hot and turning golden or the meat is thoroughly cooked.

Serve with a green salad and any leftover Beetroot risotto. Heat the remaining marinade thoroughly and serve as a sauce on the side.

You can add different sources of protein to the Mixed vegetable brochettes: tofu or haloumi can be marinated in the sauce and grilled with the vegetables. Or serve the vegetables, and the sauce, with cooked quinoa (120g/4oz is enough for two servings), or Spicy chick-peas (p.157).

Chicken brochettes

Quick country soup or Four bean salad

Sea vegetables for the soup are available in good health food shops, or use shredded spinach or kale. Save a portion of salad for lunch tomorrow, and two portions of soup.

Quick country soup

Quick country soup

ready in **30** minutes

1 medium onion, finely chopped
2 tablespoons olive oil
400g (13oz) button mushrooms, sliced
500ml (17fl oz) passata or 1x400g (13oz) can tomatoes, zapped in a blender until smooth
500ml (17fl oz) vegetable stock
1 tablespoon tomato paste
Juice ½ lemon
½ teaspoon dried Herbes de Provence
2 tablespoons dried sea vegetables or 50g (2oz) washed shredded spinach

Soften the chopped onion in the olive oil in a saucepan. Add the mushrooms and more oil if necessary. Mix well and cook for about 5 minutes. Add the passata, stock, tomato paste, lemon juice, and dried herbs and simmer for 15 minutes or so. Stir in the sea vegetables or shredded spinach and cook for a further 5–10 minutes.

Serve with a scattering of grated parmesan or hard goat's cheese over the top if you wish.

Four bean salad

ready in **10** minutes

100g (3½oz) broad beans (frozen or fresh)
100g (3½oz) green beans, topped and tailed and cut in half
100g (3½oz) mangetout or fresh petis pois
100g (3½oz) red or orange pepper
1x400g (13oz) can beans, well rinsed and drained
2 spring onions, finely chopped
A handful of chopped herbs of your choice

For the dressing:
2 tablespoons lemon juice
2 tablespoons reduced-fat fromage frais
1 tablespoon dry apple juice
1 clove garlic, crushed
1 teaspoon Dijon mustard

Steam the beans and mangetout until al dente (about 3–4 minutes). Refresh under cold running water and drain. Mix the fresh beans, petit pois, pepper, canned beans, spring onions and herbs in a bowl. Mix the dressing, pour over the salad and stir well. Season with freshly ground black pepper. Top with some crumbled feta if you like, and serve.

Duck breast or smoked tofu salad

To save time, you can make the dressing and even cook the vegetables in advance over the weekend to store in the fridge. Serves two.

ready in **30** minutes

100g (3½oz) asparagus (trimmed weight)
½ teaspoon five-spice powder
1 tablespoon olive oil
1 red pepper, cut into strips
2 medium chicory heads
(or 2 medium gem lettuce
if chicory is not in season)
2 duck breasts (approx.
200g/7oz), trimmed of
all fat, or 200–250g
(7–8oz) smoked tofu
A few toasted sesame seeds

For the dressing:
1 tablespoon olive oil
A few drops Tabasco
or a pinch of cayenne
Juice and grated zest
of ½ small orange
1 tablespoon soy sauce
2 teaspoons balsamic vinegar
A squeeze of lemon juice

Duck breast salad

Preheat the oven to 200°C/400°F/gas mark 6. Snap the tough ends off the asparagus shoots and cut the shoots in two lengths (or use asparagus tips). Mix the five-spice powder and a grinding of fresh black pepper with a tablespoon of olive oil. Put the asparagus in a small roasting pan, pour over the oil mix. Coat the asparagus in the oil. Cook in the oven for 5 minutes. Add the peppers, coat them and cook for another 5–10 minutes. The vegetables should be hot, but still with a bite.

Break up the chicory or lettuce and arrange in two shallow bowls. Mix the dressing ingredients in a small bowl.

If using duck, lightly oil a hot griddle and quickly cook the duck breasts – they should be brown on the outside and just pink on the inside. When cooked, slice the breasts into four or five slices. (If you prefer, cook the duck breasts under a grill or on a gentle barbecue.)

If using tofu, toss the tofu in a little olive oil and lightly brown, preferably under a grill.

Divide the asparagus and pepper mix over the chicory or gem lettuce, top with the duck breasts or tofu, drizzle with the dressing, sprinkle some sesame seeds over the top and serve.

Butter beans in tapenade with vegetables

Use a variety of green vegetables, such as French beans, runner beans, mangetout and asparagus, for this recipe. Serves two.

ready in 30 minutes

1 tablespoon olive oil
1 small onion, chopped
150g (5oz) small mushrooms, sliced (chestnut or exotic mushrooms add a more interesting flavour)
8 cherry tomatoes, halved
2 tablespoons tapenade
Juice ½ lemon
1 teaspoon soy sauce
¼ teaspoon chilli powder, or to taste – optional
1x400g (13oz) can butter beans, rinsed and drained
450g (14oz) mixed green vegetables, chopped
A few sprigs fresh coriander, chopped

Heat the olive oil in a frying pan and soften the onion for a few minutes. Add the mushrooms and tomatoes and cook for a further minute. Stir in the tapenade, lemon juice, soy sauce and chilli powder according to your preference. Tip in the butter beans and heat everything together for 3–4 minutes to combine all the flavours.

Put the mixed green vegetables in a steamer and steam them together until just cooked. Put aside one third of the vegetables for tomorrow's lunch. Serve the remainder with the butter beans and some chopped coriander scattered over the top.

If you like this recipe, you could double the quantities listed to give you a couple of extra lunchtime helpings instead of the menus suggested; serve with a sprouted seed salad.

Carrot & cardamom rice with a green leaf salad   DINNER DAY 16

You can cook the rice up to 24 hours in advance and keep it in the fridge if you think you will be pressed for time making dinner tonight. Serves two.

50g (2oz) red or brown rice
250ml (8fl oz) vegetable stock
2 tablespoons dried sea vegetables
2 hen's eggs
A little oil to cook the eggs
5 cardamom pods
1 tablespoon olive oil
1 small onion, chopped
100g (3½oz) carrot, coarsely grated
Grated rind 1 orange
Fresh parsley, chopped, to garnish

Simmer the rice in the vegetable stock for about 25 minutes, until just tender. Add the dried sea vegetables and stir for 2 minutes. If there is any liquid left, turn up the heat and boil hard until the liquid has evaporated. Set to one side.

In a non-stick pan, scramble the two eggs in a little oil. Then set the scrambled eggs to one side.

Slit each cardamom pod open, scrape the seeds into a pestle and crush with a mortar. Heat the oil in a frying pan and soften the onion for a few minutes. Add the crushed seeds and stir together, then add the grated carrot and orange rind. Cook for about five minutes until the carrot begins to soften. Stir in the cooked rice, fold in the scrambled egg, place the mix in a shallow baking dish, cover and cook for about 15 minutes in a hot oven. Serve with a garnish of parsley and a green leaf salad.

Snacks

Both these snacks will keep well in the fridge for up to five days, so if you make both recipes at the weekend you should have plenty of weekday snacks to hand.

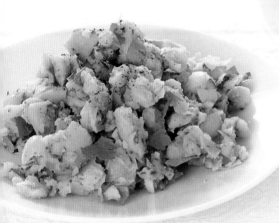

Bean & mustard mash

ready in **20** minutes

1x400g (13oz) can butter beans, drained and rinsed
Approx. 300ml (½ pint) vegetable stock
2 tablespoons olive oil
1 heaped teaspoon Dijon mustard or scant tablespoon tapenade
A small handful fresh parsley, chopped

Simmer the beans with enough vegetable stock to cover for about 15–20 minutes. Drain, reserving the stock. Put the beans in a bowl with the olive oil, mustard or tapenade and season with freshly ground black pepper. Mash the ingredients together until reasonably smooth. Stir in plenty of chopped parsley and more olive oil if necessary. Add a little of the reserved stock if the mash is too stiff. Store covered in the fridge.

Spicy chick-pea spread

ready in **10** minutes

2 tablespoons olive oil
1x400g (13oz) can chick-peas, drained and rinsed and patted dry on kitchen paper
1 teaspoon paprika

Heat the oil in a frying pan, add the chick-peas and cook, turning frequently over a medium heat until they begin to turn crispy. Tip onto a plate covered with absorbent kitchen paper to absorb any remaining oil. Put the chick-peas in a clean bowl and add the paprika. Mash the ingredients coarsely with a fork and keep in the fridge.

Brunch

Brunches are designed to be relaxed affairs, and these straightforward recipes will hopefully encourage you to sit down and enjoy your meal at leisure. All recipes serve two.

Eggs, spinach & smoked salmon

ready in **15** minutes

100g (3½oz) spinach, rinsed and cleaned well
1 generous tablespoon each reduced-fat fromage frais and live natural low-fat yoghurt
½ teaspoon grated ginger
2 hen's eggs
80g (2½oz) smoked salmon, cut into wide strips
A squeeze of lemon juice
A pinch of paprika
2 teaspoons toasted seeds *(p.51)*

If the spinach leaves are large, shred them coarsely. Steam for about 5 minutes until limp. Drain well and keep warm.

Combine the fromage frais, yoghurt and ginger. Poach the eggs as you like them.

Combine the smoked salmon and spinach with the lemon juice and season with freshly ground black pepper. Divide onto two plates. Top each with a poached egg and spoon over the yoghurt mixture. Sprinkle over the paprika and seeds.

Serve with pitta bread or a carbohydrate of your choice.

Smoked salmon pasta

ready in **20** minutes

100g (3½oz) corn pasta shells
A drizzle of olive oil
A drizzle of lemon juice
50ml (2fl oz) reduced-fat fromage frais
50ml (2fl oz) live natural low-fat yoghurt
1 tablespoon olive oil
100g (3½oz) smoked salmon
A small bunch fresh dill, chopped

Cook the pasta according to the instructions on the packet. Once cooked, strain and toss in a little olive oil and lemon juice.

Combine the fromage frais and yoghurt with the olive oil.

Cut the smoked salmon into strips. Combine the salmon with the pasta and yoghurt mix. Season with freshly ground black pepper and lemon juice to taste. Stir in the chopped dill, divide onto two plates and serve while warm.

Turkey skewers with lime & basil salsa

ready in **30** minutes

150–200g (5–7oz) boneless turkey
2 medium courgettes, cut lengthways into thin slices
2 red peppers, cut into 20 chunks

For the marinade:
2 teaspoons five-spice paste
Juice and zest 1 lime
2–3cm (¾-1in) fresh ginger, grated
2 cloves garlic, crushed
1 tablespoon olive oil
2 teaspoons sesame oil

For the salsa:
A small handful fresh basil, chopped
1 small green onion
½ yellow pepper
1 garlic clove
2 tablespoons olive oil
Juice and zest ½ lime

Mix the marinade in a bowl, cut the turkey into 16 even-sized chunks and add to the marinade. Leave for at least half an hour in the fridge. Blitz the salsa ingredients in the food processor for a few seconds.

Partly wrap a piece of meat in a courgette slice, then alternately thread the peppers and wrapped meat onto 4 soaked wooden skewers. Cook on a griddle or barbecue for 15 minutes over a medium heat. Serve with the salsa, a green salad and your choice of carbohydrate.

Deluxe omelette

ready in 25 minutes

2 tablespoons white wine
2 tablespoons water
½ teaspoon Thai fish sauce
A small handful fresh tarragon sprigs, chopped
100g (3½oz) salmon fillet
3 tablespoons pinenuts
100g (3½oz) fresh asparagus (weight after snapping off the tough end of the stalk)
4 tablespoons reduced-fat fromage frais
Juice and rind ½ lime
4 hen's eggs
4 tablespoons live natural low-fat yoghurt
A little olive oil to cook the eggs

Pour the wine, water and fish sauce into a pan and add half the tarragon. Bring to the boil and put the salmon in, skin side down. Lower the heat to a gentle simmer and cook for 10 minutes or so until the salmon is just cooked through. Lift the fish from the pan, remove the skin and coarsely flake the fish.

Toast the pinenuts in a dry pan over a medium heat, tossing frequently, until they are brown on all sides.

Steam the asparagus until just cooked – about 5–6 minutes. Cut each asparagus stalk into 3 pieces.

Mix the fromage frais, lime juice and rind together in a bowl. Gently fold in the asparagus and fish.

To make the omelettes, beat the eggs, yoghurt and remaining tarragon in a bowl. Season with freshly ground black pepper and use half the mixture to make the first omelette.

Heat a little oil in a frying pan, pour in the egg mix and cook over a medium heat. When the omelette is set underneath, but still soft on top, spread half the filling on one half of the omelette, sprinkle half the nuts on top, and then carefully fold the plain half of the omelette over the filling. Leave to cook for a few more seconds, then lift it out and keep it warm in the oven while you cook the second omelette. Then serve.

week 3
day 17

Breakfast

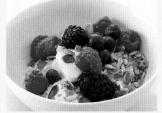

Hot lemon & ginger drink *(p.42)*

Cereal or ham breakfast

Cereal recipes are listed on pages 42, 44, 48, 50, 52 and 84; see page 76 for a ham breakfast recipe.

Morning snack

Choose either:

250ml (8oz) Red energy juice *(right)* or Energizer juice *(p.87)*, and 1 oatcake spread with your choice of topping *(below)*

OR

2 oatcakes or rye biscuits with your choice of topping:

- [ ] Crab meat spread *(see recipe, below)*
- [ ] Red lentil & turmeric spread *(p.125)*
- [ ] Sweet potato & goat's cheese topping *(p.125)*

Crab meat spread

2 tablespoons crab meat (canned or fresh)
1 tablespoon low-fat fromage frais
A good squeeze of lemon juice
A little chopped parsley, coriander or rocket (if you have some to hand)

Mix all the ingredients together and spread on the oatcakes or rye biscuits.

Lunch

Soup or tuna salad & your choice of carbohydrate

1 portion of Quick country soup reserved from day 13 or

½ remaining can of tuna (from lunch yesterday) with a mixed salad

Your choice of dressing *(pp.143,145,147)*

Your choice of carbs: 1 slice of rye or wholemeal bread or 2 oatcakes, rice cakes or rye biscuits

Heat the soup thoroughly and serve, or mix the remainder of the tuna with some salad vegetables and serve with your choice of dressing and carbohydrate.

The Food Doctor

Tip for the day ...

Soak 8 dried apricots overnight in water if you want to make tomorrow afternoon's Digestive booster smoothie.

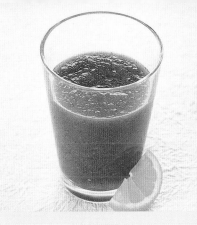

Afternoon snack

Choose either:

250ml (8oz) Vegetable smoothie (if you have portion 2 leftover from yesterday) or Apple & mint smoothie *(p.85)*

OR

2 oatcakes or rye biscuits with your choice of topping:

☐ Banana & fromage frais spread *(below)*

☐ Sweet potato & goat's cheese topping *(p.125)*

Banana & fromage frais spread

½ banana, mashed
1 tablespoon reduced-fat fromage frais
1 teaspoon sesame seeds

Mix the ingredients together and spread on the biscuits.

Dinner

Courgettes in chick-pea sauce with quinoa & salad *(p.118)*

This dish, like all the dinners on the plan, includes low-saturated fat protein and encourages you to prepare vegetables in a new and fresh way.

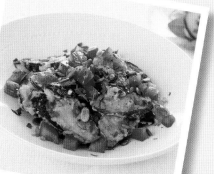

Morning snack recipe

Raw food always offers a greater level of nutrients, so this juice helps to provide you with a boost of nutritious energy. This recipe should make enough for two snacks.

Red energy juice

100ml (3½fl oz) carrot juice
75ml (3fl oz) dry apple juice
150g (5oz) cucumber
1 medium tomato
50g (2oz) red pepper
Juice 1 lemon

Put all the ingredients in a food processor and blitz for a few seconds until mixed.

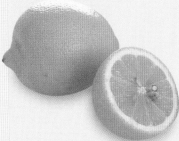

week 3
day 18

Breakfast

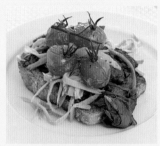

Hot lemon & ginger drink *(p.42)*

Cereal or ham breakfast

Cereal recipes are listed on pages 42, 44, 48, 50, 52 and 84; see page 76 for a ham breakfast recipe.

Morning snack

Choose either:

250ml (8oz) Red energy juice *(p.103)* **and 1 oatcake generously spread with your choice of topping** *(below)*

OR

2 oatcakes or rye biscuits spread with your choice of topping:

- [ ] Red lentil & turmeric spread *(p.125)*
- [ ] Sweet potato & goat's cheese topping *(p.125)*
- [ ] Crab meat spread *(p.102)*
- [ ] Tomato & bean mash *(below)*

Tomato & bean mash

12 cherry tomatoes
1 clove garlic, crushed
1 tablespoon olive oil
2 tablespoons barlotti beans
A little balsamic vinegar

Put the tomatoes and garlic in a roasting dish and drizzle the oil over the top. Roast in the oven at 200°C/400°F/gas mark 6 for about 15 minutes. Mix in the beans and roughly break up. Add a dash of balsamic vinegar and pile onto the oatcakes, rye biscuits or a piece of wholemeal toast.

Lunch

Carrot & cardamom rice with salad & your choice of carbohydrate

1 portion carrot and cardamom rice reserved from dinner, day 16
1 mixed salad or sprouted seeds
A little olive oil
A squeeze of lemon juice
Your choice of carbs: 1 slice of rye or wholemeal bread or 2 oatcakes, rice cakes or rye biscuits

Put the reserved rice and salad on a plate. Drizzle with a little olive oil and the lemon juice. Serve with the carbohydrate of your choice.

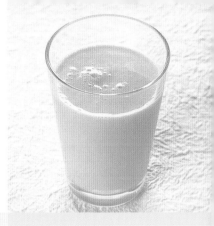

The Food Doctor

Tip for the day ...

If you want to make the Fruit compote for brunch tomorrow, soak the dried fruit in peppermint tea overnight tonight.

Afternoon snack

Choose either:

250ml (8oz) Digestive booster smoothie *(right)*

OR

2 oatcakes or rye biscuits with Chick-pea & banana spread *(p.89)* or Banana & fromage frais spread *(p.103)*

OR

Dates & fromage frais

2 teaspoons reduced-fat fromage frais
A squeeze of lime juice
2 fresh organic dates, stoned and opened
6 pumpkin seeds

Mix the fromage frais with the lime juice, divide the mixture in half and spoon into each date with the pumpkin seeds.

Dinner

Baked mushrooms & salad *(p.119)*

Save a portion for lunch tomorrow if not eating brunch

Mushrooms – and especially exotic varieties – help to boost the immune system, and are packed with B vitamins, which help to lower cholesterol.

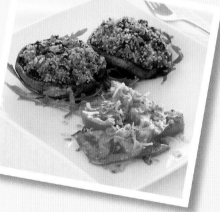

Afternoon snack recipe

The creamy, orange-tasting undertones of this luxurious smoothie give way to a lovely ginger aftertaste. The quantities listed should make 500ml (17fl oz) – enough for two smoothies. If not, top up with apple juice. Store the second portion in the fridge for tomorrow.

Digestive booster smoothie

8 dried apricots, soaked overnight in water
Juice 1 orange
Juice ½ lemon
2.5cm (1in) fresh ginger, grated
1 tablespoon sesame seeds
100ml (3½ fl oz) dry apple juice
150ml (¼ pint) live natural low-fat yoghurt

Blend all the fruits, ginger, seeds and juices together. Stir in the yoghurt. Do not sieve the smoothie as this will remove valuable fibre.

week 3
day 19

Breakfast

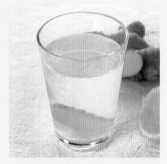

Hot lemon & ginger drink *(p.42)*

If you are having brunch today, eat a small snack at your usual breakfast time.

OR

Your choice of cereal or ham breakfast

Cereal recipes are listed on pages 42, 44, 48, 50, 52 and 84; see page 76 for a ham breakfast recipe.

Morning snack

If you are not having brunch, have 2 oatcakes or rye biscuits with your choice of spread:

☐ Crab meat spread *(p.102)*
☐ Egg & crudités *(p.88)*
☐ Red lentil & turmeric spread *(p.125)*
☐ Sweet potato & goat's cheese topping *(p.125)*
☐ The Food Doctor fresh pesto *(p.84)*
☐ Tomato & bean mash *(p.104)*

Brunch/Lunch

Brunch:
1 tonic drink *(right)*, either Fruit compote *(p.80)*, Fruit salad *(p.82)*, 1 apple or pear or 2 apricots, and your choice of brunch *(pp.100–01, 126-27)*

OR

Lunch:
Vegetable stir-fry with your choice of protein & carbohydrate

Your choice of protein, such as chicken, fish or tofu
Your choice of carbohydrate
Approx. 300g (4oz) raw vegetables per person, or 1 packet prepared vegetables
Stir-fry sauce *(p.141)*, optional

Cook the protein and prepare the carbohydrate first. Cook the vegetables in a wok over a high heat with a little water or lemon juice until al dente. If using the sauce, add it after cooking. Serve with the other prepared ingredients.

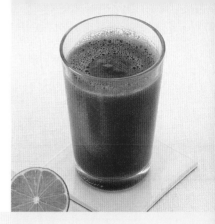

The Food Doctor

Tip for the day ...

Don't overlook the importance of a daily intake of fruits and vegetables. My plan supplies at least five portions a day.

Afternoon snack

Choose either:

250ml (8oz) Digestive booster smoothie (if you have portion 2 leftover from yesterday, day 18) or Vegetable smoothie *(p.89)*

OR

Dates & fromage frais *(p.105)*

OR

2 oatcakes or rye biscuits spread with your choice of topping:

☐ Red lentil & turmeric spread *(p.125)*

☐ Sweet potato & goat's cheese topping *(p.125)*

☐ Banana & fromage frais *(p.103)*

☐ Chick-pea & banana spread *(p.89)*

Dinner

Stir-fry curry with smoked tofu or chicken *(p.120)*

Save a portion of lentils for lunch, day 22

Spices such as turmeric have a positive effect on your blood sugar levels, and therefore on your weight.

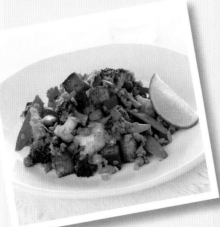

Tonics

Apple tonic

125ml (4fl oz) dry apple juice
125ml (4fl oz) water

Mix the juice and water together and serve chilled.

Cleansing tonic

125ml (4fl oz) tomato juice or passata (or 1x400g/13oz can tomatoes, blended)
125ml (4fl oz) dry apple juice
Juice ½ lemon
A dash of Tabasco sauce
2.5cm (1in) grated fresh ginger (optional)

Mix the ingredients together and serve chilled with a slice of lemon or lime.

week 3
day 20

Breakfast

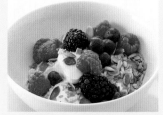

Hot lemon & ginger drink *(p.42)*

If you are having brunch today, eat a small snack at your usual breakfast time.

OR

Your choice of cereal or ham breakfast

Cereal recipes are listed on pages 42, 44, 48, 50, 52 and 84; see page 76 for a ham breakfast recipe.

Morning snack

If you are not having brunch, have 2 oatcakes or rye biscuits with your choice of spread:

- ☐ Crab meat spread *(p.102)*
- ☐ Red lentil & turmeric spread *(p.125)*
- ☐ Sweet potato & goat's cheese topping *(p.125)*
- ☐ The Food Doctor fresh pesto *(p.84)*
- ☐ Tomato & bean mash *(p.104)*

Brunch/Lunch

Brunch:
1 tonic drink *(p.107)*, either Fruit compote *(p.80)*, Fruit salad *(p.82)*, 1 apple or pear or 2 apricots, and your choice of brunch *(pp.100–01, 126-27)*

OR

Lunch:
Your choice of protein, vegetables and carbohydrate

"For brunch I had the Egg, spinach and smoked salmon – a wonderfully tasty, filling meal"

Chris

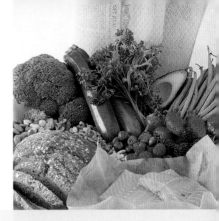

The Food Doctor

Tip for the day ...

Aim to add one new food to your diet every week to benefit from a wide variety of flavours as well as nutrients.

Afternoon snack

Choose either:

250ml (8oz) Vegetable smoothie *(p.89)* or High-energy smoothie *(p.77)*

OR

Dates & fromage frais *(p.105)*

OR

2 oatcakes or rye biscuits spread with your choice of topping:

☐ Banana & fromage frais spread *(p.103)*

☐ Chick-pea & banana spread *(p.89)*

☐ Red lentil & turmeric spread *(p.125)*

☐ Sweet potato & goat's cheese topping *(p.125)*

Dinner

Leek & potato soup or Salade niçoise

Save a portion of soup or salad for lunch tomorrow

Leeks and potatoes both have cleansing properties, while fresh tuna and eggs are ideal forms of lean protein.

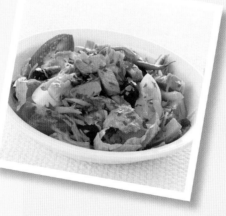

Eat a wide variety of food

The foods we eat have the greatest impact on our outward appearance and our inner energy levels, so it's vital that we eat a wide variety of food to reap the nutritional benefits.

Most of us tend to limit the range of foods we buy to those we feel comfortable eating – which can then lead to boredom and a desire to reach for fast food, processed snacks and takeaways.

One of the main aims of this plan is to encourage you to eat as many healthy foods as possible: all the recipes include nutrient-dense foods such as wholegrains, beans, pulses, nuts, seeds, oily fish and fresh seasonal vegetables. Some or most of the foods listed in this plan may be new to you, but keep trying them and you'll soon enjoy eating them. Eat a wide variety of food is Principle 3 of The Food Doctor principles *(pp.136–37)*.

week 3
day 21

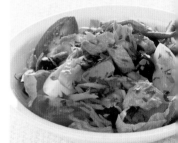

Breakfast

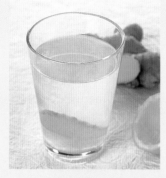

Hot lemon & ginger drink *(p.42)*

Cereal or ham breakfast

Cereal recipes are listed on pages 42, 44, 48, 50, 52 and 84; see page 76 for a ham breakfast recipe.

"We are all sitting down as a family to eat breakfast now"

Rachael

Morning snack

Choose either:

250ml (8oz) Red energy juice *(p.103)*, Energizer juice *(p.87)*, and 1 oatcake spread with your choice of topping *(below)*

OR

2 oatcakes or rye biscuits spread with your choice of topping:

- [ ] Crab meat spread *(p.102)*
- [ ] Classic guacamole *(p.80)*
- [ ] Home-made houmous *(p.46)*
- [ ] Red lentil & turmeric spread *(p.125)*
- [ ] Sweet potato & goat's cheese topping *(p.125)*
- [ ] The Food Doctor fresh pesto *(p.84)*
- [ ] Tomato & bean mash *(p.104)*

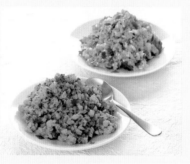

To make these snacks, see page 125

Lunch

Soup or salad & your choice of carbohydrate

1 portion Leek & potato soup or Salade niçoise reserved from dinner, day 20

2 tablespoons canned beans

Your choice of carbs: 1 slice of rye or wholemeal bread or 2 oatcakes, rice cakes or rye biscuits

Heat the soup thoroughly, or add some extra vegetables and tuna to the salad if needed, and serve with your choice of carbohydrate.

The Food Doctor

Tip for the day ...

The most colourful fruits and vegetables supply an abundance of antioxidants, so try to buy this sort of fresh produce often.

Afternoon snack

Choose either:

250ml (8oz) High-energy smoothie *(p.77)*, **Vegetable smoothie** *(p.89)* or **Digestive booster smoothie** *(p.105)*

OR

2 oatcakes or rye biscuits spread with your choice of topping:

☐ Banana & fromage frais spread *(p.103)*

☐ Chick-pea & banana spread *(p.89)*

☐ Classic guacamole *(p.80)*

☐ Red lentil & turmeric spread *(p.125)*

☐ Sweet potato & goat's cheese topping *(p.125)*

Dinner

Salmon cakes or Egg noodles with vegetables *(p.122)*

If you have the time tonight, substitute the steamed vegetables for a Coconut stir-fry *(p.178)*. Read the recipe first to check for any extra ingredients to buy.

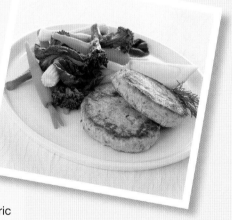

Eat protein with complex carbohydrates

Combining lean proteins such as chicken or fish with complex carbohydrates (that is, vegetables and wholegrains such as brown rice and rye bread) in the correct proportions at every meal ensures that your body receives a steady flow of energy, as the body converts these foods into glucose relatively slowly. Complex carbs also contain plenty of fibre, which promotes good digestive health.

When we think of carbohydrates, we tend to think of starchy foods such as potatoes and white rice. These foods are broken down more quickly, so it's important to avoid them.

Eat protein with complex carbohydrates is the first of The Food Doctor principles *(pp.136–37)*.

week 3
day 22

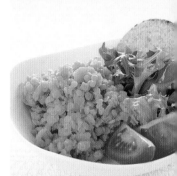

Breakfast

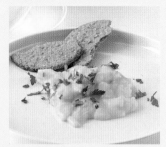

Hot lemon & ginger drink *(p.42)*

Cereal, egg or ham breakfast

Cereal recipes are listed on pages 42, 44, 48, 50, 52 and 84; egg recipes are on pages 46 and 78; see page 76 for a ham breakfast recipe.

Morning snack

Choose either:

250ml (8oz) Red energy juice *(p.103)* or Kick-start superjuice *(p.79),* and 1 oatcake spread with your choice of topping *(below)*

OR

2 oatcakes or rye biscuits spread with your choice of topping:

- [ ] Crab meat spread *(p.102)*
- [ ] Feta cheese & roast pepper spread *(below)*
- [ ] Red lentil & turmeric spread *(p.125)*
- [ ] Sweet potato & goat's cheese topping *(p.125)*
- [ ] Tomato & bean mash *(p.104)*

Feta cheese & roast pepper spread

50g (2oz) roast pepper slices (from a jar)
50g (2oz) feta cheese
A few sprigs parsley

Chop the peppers finely. Combine all the ingredients in a bowl, season with freshly ground black pepper and mash roughly with a fork.

Lunch

Tomatoes with lentils

2 sliced tomatoes
1 portion reserved lentils from dinner, day 19
1 handful green leaves
Your choice of dressing *(pp.143,145,147)*
Your choice of carbs: 1 slice of rye or wholemeal bread or 2 oatcakes, rice cakes or rye biscuits

Arrange the ingredients on a plate, drizzle over a little of your chosen dressing and serve with your choice of carbohydrate.

"I'm beginning to feel more confident about picking sensible foods to eat"

Karen

The Food Doctor

Tip for the day ...

If you are taking lunch to work tomorrow, cook a sweet potato tonight and cut it into bite-size chunks once it has cooled.

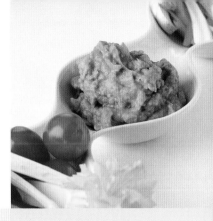

Afternoon snack

Choose either:

250ml (8oz) Digestive booster smoothie (if you have portion 2 leftover from yesterday) or Apple & mint smoothie *(p.85)*

OR

Dates & fromage frais *(p.105)*

OR

2 oatcakes or rye biscuits spread with your choice of topping:

- [ ] Banana & fromage frais spread *(p.103)*
- [ ] Chick-pea & banana spread *(p.89)*
- [ ] Classic guacamole *(p.80)*
- [ ] Feta cheese & roast pepper spread *(see recipe, left)*
- [ ] Red lentil & turmeric spread *(p.125)*
- [ ] Sweet potato & goat's cheese topping *(p.125)*

Dinner

Spicy roast ratatouille with fish or white cheese *(p.123)*

For extra flavour, add some chopped fresh herbs – whatever you have to hand or needs using up from the fridge – just before serving this dish.

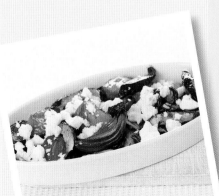

Eat fat to lose fat

There's a clear distinction between essential fats and saturated fat. The body needs essential fats in order to function properly. Foods such as avocados, nuts, oily fish, and cold-pressed oils all provide these necessary fats.

Saturated fat, on the other hand, is a non-essential fat: the body doesn't need it, even though we often find ourselves craving foods, such as crisps, that contain saturated fat.

By cutting out saturated fats and including more essential fats in your diet, you can enjoy the satisfaction that comes with eating healthy foods containing fat and minimize any cravings for unhealthy foods. Eat fat to lose fat is principle 10 of the 10 Food Doctor principles *(pp.136–37)*.

week 3
day 23

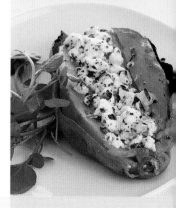

Breakfast

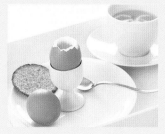

Hot lemon & ginger drink *(p.42)*

Cereal, egg or ham breakfast

Cereal recipes are listed on pages 42, 44, 48, 50, 52 and 84; egg recipes are on pages 46 and 78; see page 76 for a ham breakfast recipe.

Morning snack

Choose either:

250ml (8oz) Red energy juice *(p.103)*, or Energizer juice *(p.87)*, and 1 oatcake spread with your choice of topping *(below)*

OR

2 oatcakes or rye biscuits spread with your choice of topping:

- [ ] Bean & mustard mash *(p.99)*
- [ ] Classic guacamole *(p.80)*
- [ ] Crab meat spread *(p.102)*
- [ ] Feta cheese & roast pepper spread *(p.112)*
- [ ] Home-made houmous *(p.46)*
- [ ] Red lentil & turmeric spread *(p.125)*
- [ ] Reduced-fat fromage frais & peppers *(p.76)*
- [ ] Spicy chick-pea spread *(p.99)*
- [ ] Sweet potato & goat's cheese topping *(p.125)*
- [ ] The Food Doctor fresh pesto *(p.84)*
- [ ] Tomato & bean mash *(p.104)*

Lunch

Sweet potato with cottage cheese & spring onions

1 medium sweet potato
Your choice of dressing *(pp.143,145,147)*
2 tablespoons cottage cheese
2 spring onions, diced
1 handful green leaves
4 cherry tomatoes

Bake the sweet potato in the oven for 15–20 minutes at 180°C/350°F/gas mark 4. If you cooked the sweet potato last night, drizzle a little dressing over the dish before serving it.

Arrange the sweet potato on a plate, spoon over the cottage cheese, scatter the spring onions over the top and serve with the leaves and tomatoes on the side.

The Food Doctor

Tip for the day ...

Keep your choice of fruit and vegetables seasonal: feel free to substitute any vegetables with whatever is in season.

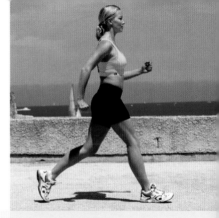

Afternoon snack

Choose either:

250ml (8oz) Apple & mint smoothie (if you have a portion leftover from yesterday)

OR

2 oatcakes or rye biscuits spread with your choice of topping:

- [ ] Sweet potato & goat's cheese topping *(p.125)*
- [ ] Banana & fromage frais *(p.103)*
- [ ] Chick-pea & banana spread *(p.89)*
- [ ] Feta cheese & roast pepper spread *(p.112)*

Dinner

Chicken or vegetarian burgers & salad *(p.124)*

To grind the seeds for the vegetarian burgers, use a blender or coffee grinder; the flat blades of a food processor may not grind the seeds finely enough.

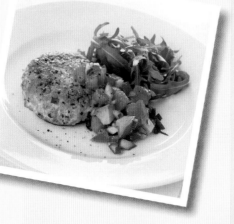

Health check

Now that you've reached the end of week 3 you should be aware of some or all of the following improvements in your health and well-being:

- [ ] Increased energy
- [ ] Falling asleep more easily
- [ ] Restful, undisturbed sleep
- [ ] More alert on waking
- [ ] No more headaches
- [ ] Less irritable
- [ ] Thicker, healthier hair
- [ ] Stronger nails
- [ ] Clearer skin
- [ ] Sparkly eyes
- [ ] Improved digestion

Don't worry if you haven't experienced many of these effects yet: you may well find that it's in week 4 that you'll begin to feel your absolute best.

Week 3 diary

Now that you've moved on to week 3, you may find yourself wanting to return to some recipes that you've enjoyed. Note down any adaptations you make to these recipes and on which days you've eaten them. Record any improvements in your health too.

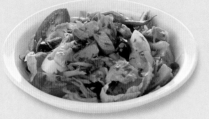

 DAY 17

What I've enjoyed eating/How do I feel?

- -
- -
- -
- -
- -
- -
- -
- -
- -
- -

DAY 20

What I've enjoyed eating/How do I feel?

- -
- -
- -
- -
- -
- -
- -
- -
- -

DAY 21

What I've enjoyed eating/How do I feel?

- -
- -
- -
- -
- -
- -
- -
- -
- -

☐ DAY 18
What I've enjoyed eating/How do I feel?

☐ DAY 19
What I've enjoyed eating/How do I feel?

☐ DAY 22
What I've enjoyed eating/How do I feel?

☐ DAY 23
What I've enjoyed eating/How do I feel?

Courgettes in chick-pea sauce, quinoa & salad | DINNER DAY 17

If you have time and want to substitute the quinoa for another protein, serve this dish with a small turkey escalope *(p.176)*. Serves two.

ready in **20** minutes

120g (4oz) quinoa (or 175g/6oz if you are cooking enough for dinner tomorrow)
250ml (8fl oz) light vegetable stock (or 300ml/12fl oz if you are cooking enough quinoa for dinner tomorrow)
2 tablespoons olive oil
400g (13oz) courgettes, sliced diagonally
1 good-sized tomato, chopped
1 handful fresh coriander or parsley, chopped
2 tablespoons toasted seeds *(p.51)*

For the sauce:
1x400g (13oz) can chick-peas, drained and rinsed (use half the can and store the rest in the fridge for snacks)
1 clove garlic, crushed
1 tablespoon lemon juice
¼ teaspoon Tabasco
½ teaspoon cumin powder
2 tablespoons live natural low-fat yoghurt

Cook the quinoa in the stock for 15 minutes or until the quinoa is soft and the liquid is absorbed. If you made extra quantities, put aside one third of the cooked quinoa for tomorrow night's supper.

Meanwhile, put all the sauce ingredients into a blender and blitz until smooth.

Heat the olive oil in a large frying pan or wok, add the courgette slices and cook until browned on both sides. Add the sauce and sizzle for a couple of minutes, until the sauce is piping hot.

Divide the courgettes between two plates, top each serving with the chopped tomatoes and herbs, and add the quinoa. Sprinkle the toasted seeds over the top of the dish and serve.

Baked mushrooms & salad

If you didn't reserve a cooked portion of quinoa from last night, tonight's supper will only take 15 minutes longer than suggested to prepare. Serves two.

ready in 25 minutes

1 portion of cooked quinoa reserved from last night (or cook 50g/2oz quinoa in 100ml/3½fl oz light stock)

4 large mushrooms (approx. 100g/3½oz per person)

1 tablespoon olive oil, plus extra to drizzle

100g (3½oz) onion, finely chopped

2 cloves garlic, crushed

8–10 black olives, stoned and finely chopped

Grated zest 1 lemon

3 good sprigs of parsley, finely chopped

A drizzle of olive oil

For the salad:

2 large slicing tomatoes

A dressing of your choice *(pp.143,145,147)*

1 spring onion, finely chopped, or sprouted seeds

If you need to cook some quinoa, gently simmer it in the stock for about 15 minutes or until it is soft and the stock is absorbed.

Cut the thick stems out of the mushrooms with a sharp knife, leaving an indentation. Chop the stems up finely.

Heat the oil in a frying pan, add the onion and soften it gently. Add the mushroom stems, garlic and olives, and cook together for a few minutes. Stir in the cooked quinoa, lemon and the parsley.

Preheat the oven to 180°C/350°F/gas mark 4. Lay the mushroom caps in a shallow baking dish, skin side down. Pile the stuffing evenly over each mushroom, patting it down firmly. Drizzle with a little olive oil, cover with foil and bake for 15–20 minutes, until the mushrooms are soft and the flavours have combined.

Serve with a salad of sliced tomatoes drizzled with a dressing of your choice, and topped with the spring onion or sprouted seeds.

Stir-fry curry with smoked tofu or chicken

DINNER DAY 19

If you want to save time tonight, substitute a can of lentils for the dried red lentils and buy a pack of ready-prepared raw vegetables. Serves two.

Stir-fry curry with smoked tofu

ready in **30** minutes

1 small onion, finely chopped

3 tablespoons olive oil

½ teaspoon curry powder

½ teaspoon turmeric powder

100g (3½oz) red lentils (or 1x400g/13oz can lentils)

200ml (l7fl oz) vegetable stock (or 50ml/2fl oz for canned lentils)

250g (8oz) mixed vegetables, chopped into bite-size pieces

1 tablespoon curry paste or powder (quantities to taste)

100g (3½oz) chicken or smoked tofu

Juice 1 lime

50ml (2fl oz) water

A small bunch fresh coriander, chopped

2 lime wedges

Soften the chopped onion in a tablespoon of olive oil, stir in the spices and cook for a couple of minutes. Add the lentils and stock. If you are using dried lentils, simmer them very gently in the stock for about 15 minutes until the lentils are soft but still keep their shape. The stock should all be absorbed. Put aside.

If you are using vegetables such as green beans, the stir-frying can be more even if the beans are blanched for a couple of minutes to start the cooking process: put in a small pan, cover with cold water, bring to the boil, simmer for 2 minutes and then drain.

Heat a tablespoon of olive oil in a wok, add the curry paste and stir. Add the chicken or tofu and stir until the chicken is cooked or the tofu is browned and has absorbed the curry flavours. Lift from the wok and put to one side. Add a further tablespoon of olive oil and a little more curry paste or powder (to taste), toss in the vegetables and stir to absorb the flavours. Add the lime juice and water and cook for a further 5–10 minutes until the vegetables are hot and al dente. Add the chicken or tofu and half the cooked lentils. Serve topped with chopped coriander and lime wedges.

Refrigerate the leftover lentils to make snacks (*p.125*).

Leek & sweet potato soup or Salade niçoise

If you want to make a vegetarian Salade niçoise, omit the tuna, use two eggs and add Spicy chick-peas *(p.157)*. Both recipes serve two.

Leek & sweet potato soup

ready in **30** minutes

1 medium onion, finely chopped
2 tablespoons olive oil
1 good-sized leek (about 200g/7oz cleaned weight), finely sliced
1 medium sweet potato (200g/7oz), peeled and coarsely grated
1 teaspoon ground cumin
1.5 litres (2 pints) well-flavoured stock
1 tablespoon dried sea vegetables (optional)
100g (3½oz) quinoa
250ml (8fl oz) light stock
1 clove garlic, peeled and left whole

Soften the onion in a tablespoon of olive oil in a large saucepan. Add the leek and potato and cook for 2 minutes. Add the cumin and pour in the stock. Simmer for 10–15 minutes. Stir in the dried sea vegetables, if using. Simmer the quinoa in the stock with the garlic. When soft (after about 15 minutes), lift out the garlic, pour the quinoa and any remaining stock into the soup and serve. You can mash the garlic into the soup if you like.

Salade niçoise

ready in **15** minutes

100g (3½oz) green or runner beans, trimmed and halved
1 fresh tuna steak (approx. 200g/7oz) or 1 can of tuna, preferably in spring water, drained
1 little gem lettuce or similar green-leaved lettuce (or use 50–100g/2–3½oz mixed green leaves)
2 medium tomatoes, cut into quarters
½ yellow pepper
1 medium carrot, coarsely grated
2 spring onions, finely sliced
6–8 black olives, pitted
Your choice of dressing *(pp.143,145,147)*
1 hard-boiled egg, shelled and quartered, or 2 eggs and Spicy chick-peas for a vegetarian option
A handful chopped fresh seasonal herbs

Steam the beans until al dente (about 3–5 minutes). If using fresh tuna, cook the fish as for day 4 *(p.59)*.

Tear the lettuce leaves coarsely into a salad bowl. Toss in the beans, tomatoes, pepper, carrot, spring onions and olives. Add the dressing and mix. Top with the egg, tuna and herbs, or two eggs, Spicy chick-peas and herbs for a vegetarian dish.

Salade niçoise

Salmon cakes or Egg noodles with vegetables

DINNER DAY 21

Choose from either the Salmon cakes or the Egg noodles for a satisfying, high-protein evening meal. Both recipes serve two.

Salmon cakes

ready in **15** minutes

150–200g (5–7oz) salmon fillet, skin removed *(p.33)*
1 medium shallot or 6 small spring onions, chopped
1 slice rye bread – about 25g (1oz)
1 egg white (reserve the yolk and add it to your scrambled egg if you are having it for breakfast tomorrow)
A squeeze of lemon juice
Zest ½ lemon
1 teaspoon tomato purée
A pinch of dried dill or ½ teaspoon chopped fresh dill
1 teaspoon olive oil
Approx. 300g (11oz) mixed vegetables per person, chopped, or 1 packet ready-prepared vegetables

Put the salmon, shallot or onions and bread into a food processor and zap to a paste. Tip into a bowl and combine with the egg white, lemon juice and zest, the purée, herbs and black pepper. Wet your hands and form two burger shapes from the mix. The thinner the cakes, the quicker they cook.

As you steam the vegetables, heat a teaspoon of olive oil in a non-stick frying pan and press the fishcakes into the oil. Cook gently for 3–4 minutes on each side – they should be golden on the outside and just cooked through the middle. Serve with wedges of lemon and the steamed vegetables.

Egg noodles

ready in **10** minutes

3 medium eggs
3 small spring onions, trimmed and finely sliced
1 tablespoon live natural low-fat yoghurt
½ teaspoon cumin
1 teaspoon olive oil

Put all the ingredients together in a bowl, season with freshly ground black pepper, and whisk well.

As you steam the vegetables, make three flat omelettes from the egg mix. Heat a little oil in a non-stick omelette pan. Pour in one third of the mix and spread it evenly around the pan. Allow to set and lightly brown on one side, flip over and brown the other side (or slip under a hot grill for a couple of minutes). Turn the omelette out onto a plate and keep it warm while you make the others. When they are all cooked, roll up each omelette and slice across to make ribbons.

Serve the egg ribbons on the steamed vegetables. Sprinkle a tablespoon of toasted mixed seeds *(p.51)* over the top if you prefer.

Salmon cakes with vegetables

Spicy roast ratatouille with fish or white cheese

DINNER DAY 22

If you use feta cheese, you can add extra protein by stirring in some chick-peas or beans before you grill the dish. Serves two.

3 cloves garlic, skin left on
1 aubergine, sliced
1 medium courgette, sliced
1 medium red onion, cut into wedges
2 beefsteak tomatoes, cut into wedges
1 teaspoon dried Herbes de Provence
½ teaspoon chilli powder, or a chopped green chilli (or in quantities to your own taste)
100ml (3½fl oz) olive oil
A squeeze of lemon juice

250–300g (8–10oz) white fish fillet (such as cod, orange roughy, halibut, haddock) or 200g (7oz) haloumi cheese or feta cheese, cubed or crumbled
2 tablespoons canned chick-peas or canned beans (optional)

Preheat the oven to 200°C/400°F/gas mark 6.

Leaving the skin on the garlic, cut off the tips. Put all the vegetables in a roasting pan together with the herbs, chilli and oil. Add a good grinding of black pepper. Cook in the hot oven for about 30 minutes, turning once or twice and adding a squeeze of lemon juice.

Squeeze a little lemon juice over the fish and cook it under a medium grill, or add the chick-peas (if using), sprinkle feta cheese over the roast vegetables, slip under a medium-hot grill for a few minutes and serve.

Spicy roast ratatouille with white cheese

Chicken or Vegetarian burgers & salad

DINNER DAY 23

If you're making Vegetarian burgers, the raw mix may appear too wet to use. However, the egg binds the ingredients together as they cook, and after the burgers are turned over.

ready in **20** minutes

Chicken burgers

300g (10oz) minced chicken or turkey (or use chicken thigh fillets and process the meat in a food processor)
2 teaspoons tamarind paste
Rind ½ lemon
½ teaspoon soy sauce
1 spring onion, chopped very finely
1 tablespoon fresh parsley or coriander, finely chopped
A large pinch chilli powder or 1 fresh chilli, chopped (optional)
1 tablespoon olive oil

Combine the minced meat with all the other ingredients except the oil in a bowl. Add a little chilli powder or fresh chopped chilli if you like it hot. Divide the mixture into 2 burgers.

Heat a tablespoon of olive oil in a frying pan, preferably non stick, over a medium-high heat. Drop in the burgers and brown one side for a couple of minutes, then turn and brown on the other side. Turn down the heat a little to prevent any burning, and cook each side for a further 4–5 minutes so that the meat is thoroughly cooked.

Serve with a green salad and a dressing of your choice *(pp.143,145,147)*.

Vegetarian burgers

200g (7oz) firm tofu
2 spring onions, shredded lengthways and finely sliced
4 shiitake mushrooms, stalks removed and finely diced (or use small brown or button mushrooms)
25g (¾oz) carrots, finely grated
2.5cm (1in) fresh ginger root, finely grated
2 teaspoons tamarind paste
1 teaspoon soy sauce
5 tablespoons mixed or toasted seeds *(p.51)*
1 tablespoon fresh parsley or coriander, finely chopped
1 hen's egg, lightly beaten
1 tablespoon olive oil

Drain the tofu and firmly pat dry using absorbent kitchen paper. Combine all the ingredients except the oil in a bowl and mix. Divide into 4 burgers.

Heat a frying pan, preferably non stick, with a little olive oil over a medium-high heat. Brown each side for about 4 minutes, turning only once. Use a spatula to pat the mixture together after you turn each burger over.

Serve with a green salad and a dressing of your choice *(pp.143,145,147)*.

Snacks

These snacks are tasty, filling and high in protein. They're also versatile enough to be used as a side dish with a meal if you wish. Keep in the fridge for up to five days.

Red lentil & turmeric spread

1 tablespoon olive oil
1 medium onion, finely chopped
1 clove garlic, chopped
1 bay leaf
2 teaspoons ground turmeric
2 teaspoons curry powder
½ teaspoon chilli paste, or 1 small fresh chilli, chopped
2 teaspoons black mustard seeds
½ teaspoon cumin seeds
150g (5oz) red lentils
300ml (½ pint) vegetable stock
1–2 tablespoons fresh coriander, finely chopped

Heat the oil in a small saucepan and gently cook the onion, garlic and bay leaf until the onion is soft, but not coloured. Stir in the turmeric, curry powder, chilli paste or fresh chilli, and mustard and cumin seeds and cook gently for 3–4 minutes to allow the onion to absorb the flavours.

Add the lentils and stock. Stir and simmer gently for about 15 minutes until the lentils are very tender and the stock is absorbed. Mash the ingredients coarsely, stir in the fresh coriander and season with some freshly ground black pepper. Keep covered in the fridge.

Sweet potato & goat's cheese topping

200g (7oz) sweet potato, peeled and coarsely chopped
2 garlic cloves in their skins, tips chopped off
1 tablespoon olive oil
75g (2½oz) soft goat's cheese, roughly cubed
Lemon juice, to taste
1–2 tablespoons fresh coriander, chopped

Preheat the oven to 350C/180F/gas mark 4.

Put the chopped sweet potato and garlic cloves in a baking dish. Toss the pieces in the oil, cover the dish and put it in the preheated oven. Bake for about 25 minutes, or until the sweet potato pieces are soft. Allow to cool, then squeeze the soft garlic cloves out of their skins and tip into a bowl with the sweet potato. Add the goat's cheese and mash together until well blended, but not reduced to a smooth purée. Add the lemon juice, season with freshly ground black pepper to taste and add the fresh coriander. Store, covered, in the fridge.

Brunch

These brunch recipes are all quick and easy to make. Buckwheat wraps, a great form of carbohydrate, are a tasty alternative to toast, and versatile enough to be used for other meals too. All recipes serve two.

Poached egg country style

ready in **10** minutes

2 hen's eggs
1 tablespoon olive oil
120g (4oz) mushrooms, sliced (brown mushrooms give a better flavour)
2 medium tomatoes, sliced
100g spinach, washed and shredded
2 slices of wholemeal or rye toast

Heat a large frying pan of water and cook the poached eggs as you like them. Heat the olive oil in a frying pan, add the mushrooms and cook over a gentle heat until they are soft and just turning brown. Add the tomatoes and spinach. Heat until the spinach has wilted and the tomatoes are hot.

Heap the mushroom mix onto lightly buttered toast and top with the poached eggs. Season with a good grinding of black pepper and serve.

Mixed grill wrap

ready in **20** minutes

2 medium tomatoes, quartered
2 medium mushrooms, quartered
1 medium pepper (yellow makes a nice contrast in colour), cut into thin slices
2 tablespoons olive oil
100g (3½oz) liver (chicken, calf, lamb or venison)

For the buckwheat wraps:
100g (3½oz) buckwheat flour
1 large hen's egg
300ml (½ pint) milk and water mixed (or all water)
½ teaspoon dried Herbes de Provence
1 teaspoon olive oil

For the sauce:
3 teaspoons soy sauce
3 teaspoons Dijon mustard
1 tablespoon lemon juice

To make the wraps, put the flour into a large bowl. Make a well in the middle and break the egg into the well. Using a whisk, gradually add the fluid, whisking until the mix is like thin cream. Add the herbs and season with black pepper.

Heat the oil in an omelette or pancake pan. Add about 75ml (3fl oz) of the mixture and cook for a few minutes. Flip over and brown the other side. When cooked, turn onto an upturned plate, cover with another plate and make the other wraps. The mix should make 4 wraps; freeze the excess wraps for up to one month, or store in the fridge for up to two days.

Put the tomatoes, mushrooms and pepper into a grill pan and toss them in a tablespoon of olive oil. Season with freshly ground black pepper. Grill under a medium grill for about 10 minutes, turning frequently, until the vegetables are soft.

Heat another tablespoon of oil in a frying pan and gently cook the liver for 4–6 minutes, depending on the thickness of the meat. It should be nicely brown on the outside, but still slightly pink in the middle. Once cooked, cut the liver into several small slices. Mix the sauce ingredients together and pour into a jug.

Put a wrap back in the pan, heat one side gently, turn over and fill half the wrap with half of the grilled vegetables. Top with half of the liver and pour over a little of the sauce. Fold the wrap in half and leave in the pan for a couple of minutes to heat through. Make another mixed-grill wrap and serve.

Warm lentil & poached egg salad

ready in 15 minutes

1 tablespoon olive oil
1 small onion, finely chopped
1 small carrot, finely chopped
1 small celery stick, finely chopped
1 red pepper, deseeded and roughly chopped
100g (3½oz) flat mushrooms, sliced
150g (5oz) canned puy or brown lentils, drained and rinsed
2 hen's eggs
50g (2oz) fresh spinach
1 tablespoon balsamic vinegar

Heat the oil in a saucepan and soften the onion, carrot, and celery over a low heat. Cook for 5 minutes. Add the pepper and mushrooms and cook for a further 5 minutes.

Add the lentils to the pan. Stir all the ingredients together and allow the lentils to heat through thoroughly.

Heat a large frying pan of water and poach the eggs. While the eggs cook, add the spinach to the lentil mix and cook until the spinach has wilted.

Stir in the vinegar, spoon into two bowls and season with freshly ground black pepper. Top each bowl with a poached egg and serve.

Diet Club diaries

Three weeks on from the start of The Food Doctor Diet plan, and our Diet Club members are really getting into the swing of their new lifestyle. Everyone is reporting noticeable improvements in their health and eating habits.

Chris says "The last two weeks have given me much more flexibility, which has been welcome. I feel amazing, full of energy and life. My body is responding well to all this nutrition. I've noticed my eating patterns are changing. For instance, I tend to delay getting on with my work by eating. Previously I would have had chocolate or biscuits, but now I have a Food Doctor snack or drink water or herb teas. I feel far more in control of what I eat than I have ever done before. I am afraid of trying the 80:20 rule (p.137), as I love chocolate and might lack self-discipline.

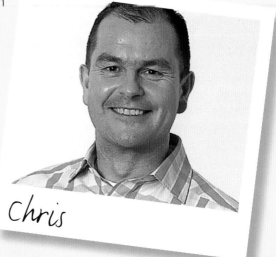

Chris

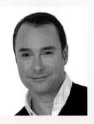

Ian says "Chris seems to have really enjoyed following the second and third weeks of the plan, and he has appreciated how much easier things can become when the plan is more adaptable and less prescriptive. I am pleased to read that Chris is already experiencing so many health benefits, and although I repeatedly hear from my own clients about how well they are feeling and sleeping, and how their energy levels are much improved, it's always a pleasure to see how well my plan works in action with other individuals. Chris has identified particular eating patterns and habits in the way that he approaches different activities – such as using sugary, starchy food as an excuse to avoid starting work – but now that he feels so much more positive about knowing how he can control his attitude to food, even this potentially difficult issue has significantly improved. It should become even easier for him to continue to manage these sorts of situations in the future. It's of particular interest to me that Chris is still thinking in terms of eating chocolate with needing to acquire a lot of self-discipline. I am confident that by significantly reducing the desire to overeat what are seen as "bad foods" on this plan, you won't need to make a conscious effort to be self-controlled. By keeping a check on his glucose levels, I am confident that Chris will achieve a happy balance using the 80:20 rule."

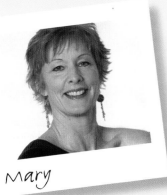

Mary

Mary says "By the end of week 2 my energy levels had really picked up, and I've slept much better. As week 3 got busier with work I found it a challenge to find time to eat snacks. When my old cravings returned I realized how important it is to keep to the plan."

Ian says "Mary experiences lows in blood glucose/sugar quite keenly, so it's essential that she snacks in between meals without fail. When work is busy, it's tempting to just keep on going, but Mary should bear in mind that she really needs the fuel from this food to provide her with consistent energy."

Joan says "I'm feeling more alert and I'm sleeping better, but I found I was hungry between my lunch and afternoon snacks. I think it's because Jon and I have been sharing the portion we reserved from our evening meals rather than making a little extra."

Ian says "It's good to see that Joan has recognized why she is hungry, as she can now see how a small change can have a profound benefit. The second and third weeks allow far more freedom than the first week, and so Joan can change things around to suit her appetite and lifestyle."

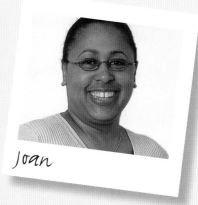

Joan

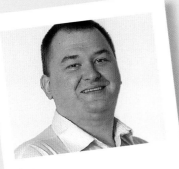

Jon

Jon says "At first I struggled on my night shifts, which may be due to having breakfast, and then dinner straight after so as to eat with Joan. This left two snacks and lunch for the rest of the night."

Ian says "Working night shifts is never easy, but combining it with wanting to eat with your partner is especially difficult. Jon was eating two meals close together, then trying to last on a smaller amount of food than is appropriate for someone of his stature. Spreading small meals evenly through the day – or night – would have been a much better method."

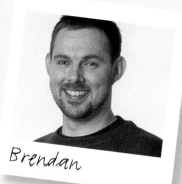

Brendan

Brendan says "A stone lost! I feel really good about that. Although I don't want to obsess about weighing myself, it's one of those things that gives a tangible sense of progress and boosts my confidence."

Ian says "Milestones are always pleasing, but the test of a good healthy eating plan is how you feel, not the figures on the scales, so don't weigh yourself too often. Having said that, Brendan hasn't been on a weight loss plan before and this way of eating is new to him, so it's good to hear that he is excited."

Karen says "I'm sleeping really well, and am full of energy. I've been doing a lot of walking, but not much other exercise. I'm feeling more confident in my food choices, and I've got into the routine of packing enough food for the day to take to work."

Ian says "Getting into a simple routine of taking food with you for the day works wonders, and I am pleased that Karen has been planning ahead so diligently. With regard to exercise, I feel that you should do something that is practical and that you can keep on doing, so if walking for miles suits Karen's lifestyle, then that's what she should stick with."

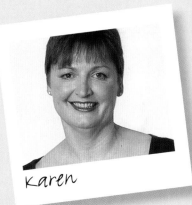

Karen

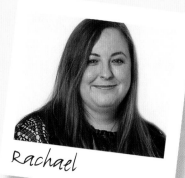

Rachael

Rachael says "Now there's more choice in the plan, thinking about each snack was hard going at first. Then I got used to it and I like the sense of control it gives me. Being with friends and family is hard: I sat in another room during one Sunday dinner."

Ian says "Moving into the second week can be daunting at first, but Rachael soon got the hang of it. It does feel good to be in control of what you eat, and Rachael should feel more confident about enjoying food with her family: she could have had some meat, just a couple of potatoes and lots of vegetables."

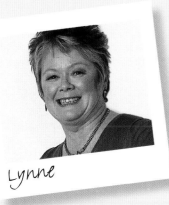

Lynne

Lynne says " I don't have time to eat before I go to work so I'm trying to follow Ian's advice and have an apple or a pear on my way out of the house and then eat my home-made muesli when I get to work."

Ian says "Having something to eat at home, even if it's only a small snack and not a proper breakfast, is a good approach to eating if you really don't have time to make breakfast. I would prefer that Lynne had a few sesame and pumpkin seeds, as well as her piece of fruit, at home. Then she would be getting some protein too, which would be ideal."

Katie says "I have been missing pizza and fresh pasta this week – they are a couple of my favourite foods. I'm starting to think that, after the plan has finished, the slightest bit of food that isn't good for me will ruin the hard work I've put in."

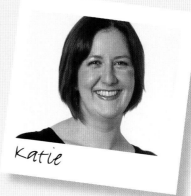

Katie

Ian says "It's quite normal for Katie to feel that some of her favourite foods could trigger old habits and undo all the hard work that she has put in. However, I suggest that Katie uses the 80:20 rule after the plan finishes, as it will help to prevent the sort of dramatic failure that is worrying her."

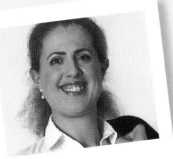

silvia

Silvia says "I've felt better than I did in week 1. I am sleeping well, but my daughter is always up at 5.30am so I feel a little irritable. One of the most positive aspects of this plan is that I'm discovering ingredients I've never tried before.

Ian says "Sleeping well is always a good sign, and feeling rested and energetic is the best way to start the day, even if you do get woken up very early! I am delighted that Silvia is enjoying trying new foods, as most of us tend to eat on auto-pilot, eating the same foods month in, month out. "

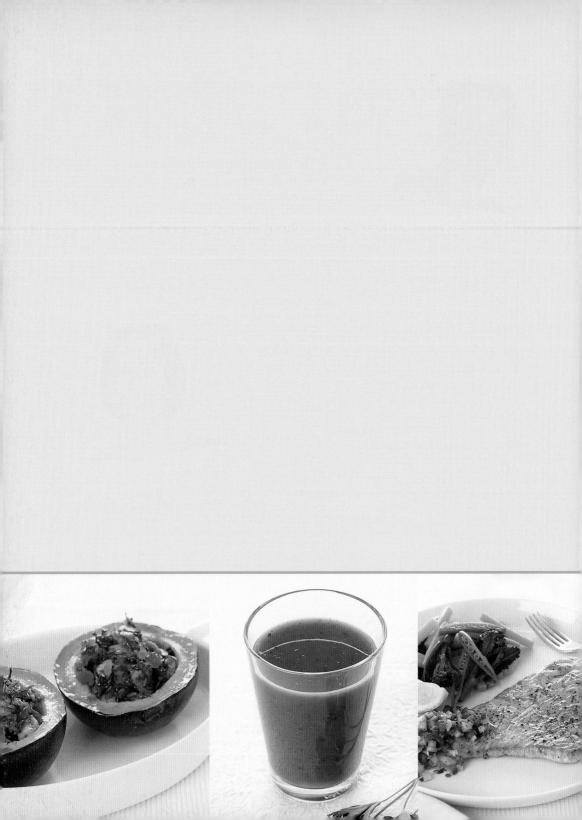

Week 4 & beyond:eat better forever

Welcome to the final week of The Food Doctor Diet plan. You may well find that this week is easier than the previous weeks because it provides you with ample choice while still providing simple yet delicious meals and snacks.

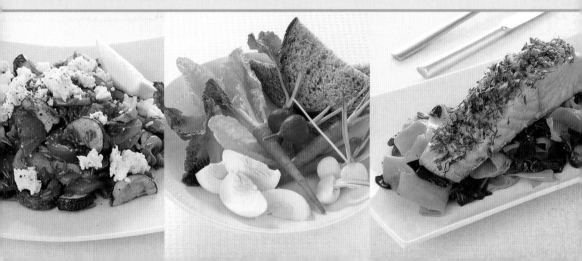

Eat better forever: Ian's advice

When you started this plan, you may have thought that the end was a long way off, but now that you are entering the final week you should be finding that my eating plan is second nature. This week is the blueprint for how you will eat in the future.

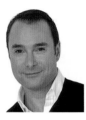

My aim has been to lead you through a month-long programme that will set you up and leave you feeling your best so you can carry on eating healthily from now on. This last week really underlines how you will be eating after this month has passed.

Week 4 differs from the previous weeks in that you have far more freedom to decide what you want to eat. It's up to you to choose which Food Doctor breakfasts, snacks and lunches you'd like each day. Despite the choices, supper recipes are still provided and this week's shopping list will help you organize yourself for these meals. Feel free to swap things around to suit yourself within the rules of combining food groups (pp.136–37).

Progress check

The Diet Club members have been doing well, and it's gratifying to read about their positive experiences. Clothes that were languishing at the backs of wardrobes because they were too small have been rescued, and everyone seems to be enjoying the compliments they are getting about how well they look. Aside from their noticeable weight loss, they are also noticing clearer, fresher-looking skin and brighter eyes. Their quality of sleep has improved and, in more than one case, they are reporting that their memory has improved. They are feeling generally more positive and confident about themselves too.

The effort involved in making meals and snacks seems to have paid off for the Diet Club members, and now that you have more freedom and choice this week, you may find that your preparation and cooking times are becoming quicker. The benefits that everyone has experienced show that the time investment has been really worthwhile.

Feel free to **swap** things around to **suit yourself** within the **rules** of the plan

Boosting your exercise routine

Now that you have more energy, you may want to exercise more, so eat a Food Doctor snack just before and after a work-out. Remember that you're not trying to burn off calories by eating too little, so if you increase your energy output, eat a little more food. This avoids creating a gap between energy intake and expenditure, which could alert the metabolic rate to a potential famine. If you don't have time to exercise, keep moving. Have a good week and enjoy this last stage of the plan.

Shopping list for week 4, days 24–30

This shopping list includes approximate quantities for seven dinner recipes only. It does not include ingredients for your choice of Food Doctor breakfasts, snacks, brunches or lunches.

This list is repeated at the end of the book for your convenience: rip out page 186 to take shopping.

- [ ] Lemons, 3
- [ ] Limes, 1
- [ ] Oranges, 1
- [ ] Broad beans, 100g (3½oz)
- [ ] Broccoli, 250g (8oz)
- [ ] Carrots, approx. 300g (10oz)
- [ ] Courgettes, medium, 2
- [ ] Fennel, 1
- [ ] Mixed raw vegetables, approx. 600g (1lb 3½oz) or equivalent weight of ready-prepared vegetables in packets
- [ ] Mixed salad ingredients: enough for 4 portions
- [ ] Mushrooms (brown), 60g (2½oz)
- [ ] Onions, medium, 1
- [ ] Peppers, red (bell, jalopeno or romano), large, 1, OR 1 jar red peppers
- [ ] Red onions, medium, 1
- [ ] Spinach fresh, 450g (15oz)
- [ ] Spring onions, 1 bunch
- [ ] Sweet potatoes, medium, 1
- [ ] Tomatoes, medium, 1
- [ ] Coriander, fresh, 1 packet
- [ ] Dill, fresh, 1 bunch
- [ ] Ginger, fresh, 1 large piece (if you have run out)
- [ ] Parsley, fresh, 1 bunch
- [ ] Rosemary, fresh, 2 sprigs
- [ ] Feta cheese, 1 packet
- [ ] Haloumi, 1 packet (if making Haloumi & mushrooms, day 25)
- [ ] Hen's eggs, 4 (plus 2 if making Ginger eggs, day 28)
- [ ] Live natural low-fat yoghurt, 1 large pot (if you have run out)
- [ ] Tofu, 1 packet (if making Tofu stir-fry, day 29)
- [ ] Chicken breasts, 2, approx. 300g (10oz) (if making Chicken stir-fry, day 29)
- [ ] Salmon fillets, 2, 200–300g (7–10oz) (if making Ginger salmon, day 28)
- [ ] White fish fillets (sole, orange roughy, cod, haddock), 200–300g (7–10oz) (if making Fish & mushrooms, day 25)
- [ ] Mixed roast peppers in oil, 250g (8oz) jar, 1
- [ ] Dry apple juice, 1 carton
- [ ] Sundried tomatoes, 60g (2½oz)
- [ ] Camargue (red) or brown risotto rice, 1 packet (if you have run out)
- [ ] Red kidney beans, 1x400g (13oz) can (if you have run out)
- [ ] Vegetable stock, 550ml (19fl oz)

DAY 27 DINNER OPTIONS

Tuscan bean soup

- [ ] Carrots, medium, 1
- [ ] Celery, 2 sticks
- [ ] Leeks, large, 1
- [ ] Onions, small, 1
- [ ] Mixed beans, 1x400g (13oz) can
- [ ] Dried sea vegetables, 1 small packet (optional)
- [ ] Raw cashews, 1 small packet (if you have run out)
- [ ] Vegetable stock, 1 litre (1¾ pints)

Mixed bean salad

- [ ] Carrot, medium, 1
- [ ] Celery, 1 stick
- [ ] Cucumber, ½
- [ ] Pepper (red/yellow/orange), 1
- [ ] Tomatoes, medium, 3
- [ ] Mixed beans, 1x400g (13oz) can
- [ ] Dried sea vegetables or seaweed, 1 small packet

10 principles

These 10 Food Doctor principles are my essential guidelines for how to eat well for the rest of your life. Don't just select certain principles: they are all vital if you want to have a healthier attitude to food. For the purposes of this month-long plan, continue to avoid Principle 8, Follow the 80:20 rule, until you have finished day 30.

1 Eat protein with complex carbohydrates

Combining these food groups in the right proportions will give you a steady flow of energy, as the body converts foods relatively slowly into glucose. This avoids triggering insulin production, so minimizing the potential for your body to store food as fat.

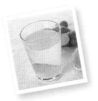

2 Stay hydrated

Drink at least 1.5 litres (3½ pints) of water a day and more in hot weather or if you are exercising. Remember, by the time you feel thirsty you are already dehydrated. After you finish The Food Doctor 30-day Diet plan, limit your alcohol and salt intake, as they dehydrate the body.

3 Eat a wide variety of food

Avoid getting stuck in a routine when you are out shopping. Most of us buy the same 10 per cent of foods for 90 per cent of the time, so try introducing two new foods to your shopping list every week.

4 Fuel up frequently

Eat the right foods little and often. By eating breakfast, lunch, dinner and regular snacks, you'll have a constant supply of energy and avoid insulin over-production, hunger, tiredness and food cravings. So although you eat more regularly at set times of the day, you still lose weight.

5 Eat breakfast

A balanced breakfast containing protein will supply you with enough fuel to help maintain energy levels and set your metabolism up for the day. Eating breakfast is fundamental to controlling your weight and feeling energetic in the long term.

6 Avoid sugar

Sugar breaks down into glucose extremely quickly, therefore contributing to fat production and weight gain. The quick, but short-lived, release that sugar gives you creates a high, and the resulting low causes hunger cravings. Avoiding sugar also helps you achieve good digestive health.

7 Exercise is essential

Healthy eating must go hand-in-hand with exercise. Exercise increases your metabolic rate – the speed at which your body uses up food as energy. Aim to fit in 30 minutes of exercise three times a week. At the very least, keep moving as much as you can.

8 Follow the 80:20 rule

It is perfectly normal to stray every now and then. If you follow the 10 Food Doctor principles for 80 per cent of the time, you can stray for the other 20 per cent without feeling guilty. This means you can enjoy social occasions and also escape the boredom and frustration associated with diet regimes.

9 Make time to eat

Try not to eat in a hurry. Taking time over a meal is beneficial to your digestive health: chewing each mouthful slowly means that your body can digest your food more effectively. Your food will also taste more satisfying as a result.

10 Eat fat to lose fat

Fat is not always the enemy. The body needs certain essential fats (omega-3 and omega-6) to function properly. It is saturated fat that you need to avoid. Include essential fats in your diet up to four or five times a week.

Build your plate

Now that you've embarked on week 4 and have even more freedom about what you can choose to eat, it's important that you get your portion sizes accurate: you need to eat the correct amount of food to sustain your energy levels perfectly.

Lunch proportions

This lunchtime meal shows the ideal ratio of protein to complex carbohydrates. The size of protein you eat should be a little smaller than the palm of your hand, while vegetables should make up the largest proportion of carbohydrates. This balance of foods should supply you with enough nutrients and energy until your mid-afternoon snack.

40%
carbohydrates
as vegetables

40% protein
as chicken

20% starchy
carbohydrates
as brown rice

Dinner ratios

If you eat before 7pm in the evening, you can include a small spoonful of starchy complex carbohydrates if you wish. However, if you eat later on in the evening, you should avoid starchy carbohydrates altogether, since you won't be using up the energy they create. This means that you should add some extra vegetables to your evening meal so that the ratios are nearer to 40 per cent protein and 60 per cent vegetables.

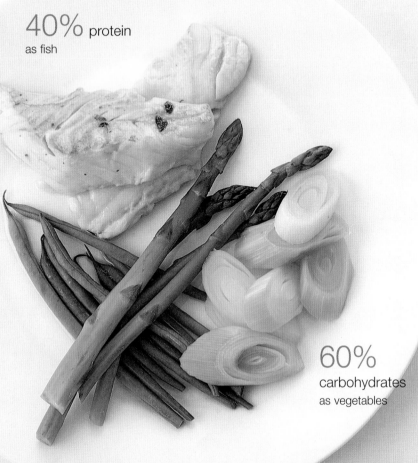

40% protein
as fish

60%
carbohydrates
as vegetables

week 4
days 24-25

Breakfast

Your choice of Food Doctor cereal or ham breakfast

Cereal recipes are listed on pp.42, 44, 48, 50, 52 and 84; a ham recipe is listed on p.76

Morning snack

Your choice of juice and 1 oatcake, or 2 oatcakes or rye biscuits, spread with a protein topping such as:

- [ ] Bean & mustard mash (p.99)
- [ ] Home-made houmous (p.46)
- [ ] Reduced-fat fromage frais & peppers (p.76)
- [ ] Spicy chick-pea spread (p.99)
- [ ] The Food Doctor fresh pesto (p.84)

Lunch

Your choice of protein, vegetables and carbohydrates (see p.150)

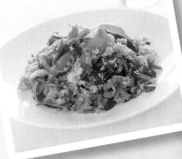

Breakfast

Your choice of Food Doctor cereal or ham breakfast

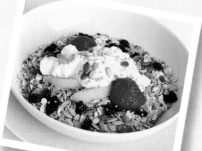

Morning snack

Your choice of juice and 1 oatcake, or 2 oatcakes or rye biscuits, spread with a protein topping such as:

- [ ] Egg & crudités (p.88)
- [ ] Flavoured no-fat soft cheese (p.42)
- [ ] Red lentil & turmeric spread (p.125)
- [ ] Sweet potato & goat's cheese topping (p.125)

Lunch

Your choice of protein, vegetables and carbohydrates (see Lunch ideas, p.150)

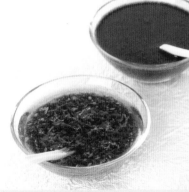

The Food Doctor

Tip for the day ...

Carry some unsalted nuts or seeds and
a piece of fruit in your bag or briefcase
so you always have an accessible snack.

Afternoon snack

Your choice of smoothie
and 1 tablespoon of
mixed seeds, or Dates &
fromage frais (p.105) or 2
oatcakes or rye biscuits,
spread with a protein
topping such as:

☐ Banana & fromage
  frais spread (p.103)

☐ Chick-pea & banana
  spread (p.89)

☐ Classic guacamole
  (p.80)

☐ Cottage cheese

Dinner

Mexican bean omelette or frittata
& salad (p.158)

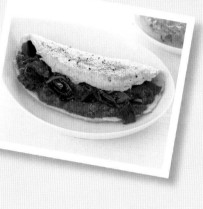

Stir-fry sauces

Making your own stir-fry
sauces is quick and easy
(bought sauces are usually
high in salt and sugar).

Fresh lime sauce

2.5cm (1in) fresh ginger, grated
1 clove garlic, crushed
Rind 1 lime, grated
4 tablespoons lime juice
2 tablespoons soy sauce
1 tablespoon balsamic vinegar
1 tablespoon olive oil

Mix all the ingredients together
and add the sauce to the stir-fry
after cooking.

Afternoon snack

Your choice of smoothie
and 1 tablespoon of
mixed seeds, or Dates
& fromage frais (p.105)
or 2 oatcakes or rye
biscuits, spread with
a protein topping
such as:

☐ Feta cheese & roast
  pepper spread (p.112)

☐ Tomato & bean mash
  (p.104)

Dinner

Fish or haloumi, mushrooms
& stir-fry (p.159)

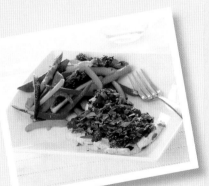

Spicy sauce

2 tablespoons five-spice paste
2 tablespoons soy sauce
1 tablespoon apple juice
1 clove garlic, crushed
1 tablespoon balsamic vinegar
1 tablespoon lemon juice

Mix all the ingredients together
and add the sauce to the stir-fry
after cooking.

week 4
days 26-27

Breakfast

If you're not having brunch, make eggs for breakfast

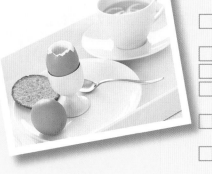

Morning snack

Your choice of juice and 1 oatcake, or 2 oatcakes or rye biscuits, spread with a protein topping such as:

- [ ] Bean & mustard mash (p.99)
- [ ] Cottage cheese
- [ ] Crab meat spread (p.102)
- [ ] Home-made houmous (p.46)
- [ ] Reduced-fat fromage frais & peppers (p.76)
- [ ] Spicy chick-pea spread (p.99)

Brunch/Lunch

See pages 100–01 and 126–27 for ideas on what to make for brunch, and pages 80–81 and 106–07 for suggestions on what to eat and drink with your main brunch dish

OR

Look at pages 150–51 for ideas of what to have for lunch

Breakfast

If you're not having brunch, choose a ham or cereal recipe for breakfast

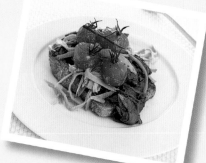

Morning snack

Your choice of juice and 1 oatcake, or 2 oatcakes or rye biscuits, spread with a protein topping such as:

- [ ] Egg & crudités (p.88)
- [ ] Flavoured no-fat soft cheese (p.42)
- [ ] Red lentil & turmeric spread (p.125)
- [ ] Sweet potato & goat's cheese topping (p.125)

Brunch/Lunch

Your choice of brunch or lunch (above)

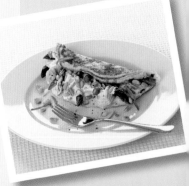

The Food Doctor

Tip for the day ...

If you're having brunch this weekend, remember to have a small snack first thing in the morning instead of breakfast.

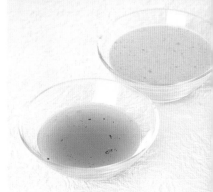

Afternoon snack

Your choice of smoothie and 1 tablespoon of mixed seeds, or Dates & fromage frais *(p.105)* or 2 oatcakes or rye biscuits, spread with a protein topping such as:

☐ Banana & fromage frais spread *(p.103)*

☐ Chick-pea & banana spread *(p.89)*

☐ Cottage cheese

☐ Classic guacamole *(p.80)*

Dinner

Mediterranean risotto *(p.160)*

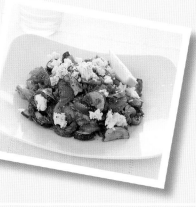

Afternoon snack

Your choice of smoothie and 1 tablespoon of mixed seeds, or Dates & fromage frais *(p.105)* or 2 oatcakes or rye biscuits, spread with a protein topping such as:

☐ Feta cheese & roast pepper spread *(p.112)*

☐ Tomato & bean mash *(p.104)*

Dinner

Tuscan bean soup or Mixed bean salad *(p.161)*

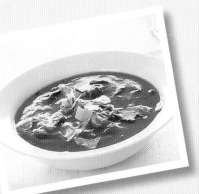

Salad dressing

Like stir-fry sauces, bought salad dressings are usually high in salt and sugar, and even saturated fat. Try this salad dressing, and also those listed on pages 145 and 147, as delicious alternatives. This recipe makes 100ml (3½fl oz). Store any extra dressing in a screw-top container in the fridge. It should keep for up to five days.

Lemon & carrot juice dressing

50ml (2fl oz) carrot juice
3 tablespoons olive oil
1 tablespoon live natural low-fat yoghurt
1 tablespoon lemon juice
½ teaspoon red chilli paste

Mix all the ingredients well, season with freshly ground black pepper and drizzle over a salad just before serving.

week 4
days 28-29

Breakfast

Your choice of Food Doctor Diet plan breakfast

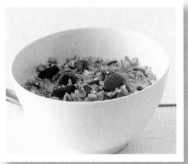

Morning snack

Your choice of juice and 1 oatcake, or 2 oatcakes or rye biscuits, spread with a protein topping such as:

- [ ] Bean & mustard mash (p.99)
- [ ] Cottage cheese
- [ ] Home-made houmous (p.46)
- [ ] Reduced-fat fromage frais & peppers (p.76)
- [ ] Spicy chick-pea spread (p.99)
- [ ] The Food Doctor fresh pesto (p.84)

Lunch

Tuscan bean soup or Mixed bean salad reserved from day 27

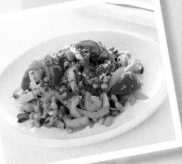

Breakfast

Your choice of Food Doctor Diet plan breakfast

Cereal recipes are listed on pages 42, 44, 48, 50, 52 and 84; egg recipes are on pages 46 and 78; see page 76 for a ham breakfast recipe.

Morning snack

Your choice of Food Doctor Diet plan snack

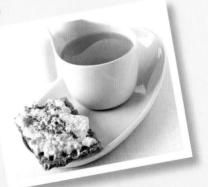

Lunch

Your choice of Food Doctor Diet plan lunch, or try this suggestion:

Baked sweet potato & steamed spinach with spicy chick-peas (p.157). Add extra steamed vegetables if necessary

Tip for the day ...

Prepare the ingredients and marinate your choice of chicken or tofu in the evening on day 28, or in the morning on day 29.

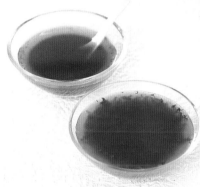

Afternoon snack

Your choice of smoothie and 1 tablespoon of mixed seeds, or Dates & fromage frais *(p.105)* or 2 oatcakes or rye biscuits, spread with a protein topping such as:

- [ ] Banana & fromage frais spread *(p.103)*
- [ ] Chick-pea & banana spread *(p.89)*
- [ ] Classic guacamole *(p.80)*

Dinner

Salmon or eggs with spinach & sweet potato *(p.162)*

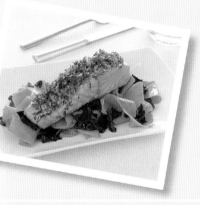

Afternoon snack

Your choice of smoothie and 1 tablespoon of mixed seeds, or Dates & fromage frais *(p.105)* or 2 oatcakes or rye biscuits, spread with a protein topping such as:

- [ ] Feta cheese & roast pepper spread *(p.112)*
- [ ] Tomato & bean mash *(p.104)*

Dinner

Chicken or tofu & broccoli stir-fry *(p.163)*

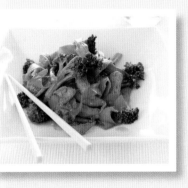

Salad dressing recipes

Store any extra salad dressing in separate screw-top containers in the fridge for up to five days.

Olive dressing

1 heaped teaspoon tapenade
4 tablespoons olive oil
2 tablespoons lemon juice
1 tablespoon orange juice

Mix all the ingredients together well. Drizzle some dressing over a salad just before serving.

Oriental dressing

3 tablespoons olive oil
1 tablespoon soy sauce
1 tablespoon lime juice
½ teaspoon five-spice paste

Mix all the ingredients together well. Drizzle some dressing over a salad just before serving.

week 4
day 30

Breakfast

Your choice of Food Doctor
Diet plan breakfast

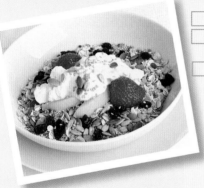

Morning snack

Your choice of juice and
1 oatcake, or 2 oatcakes or rye
biscuits, spread with a protein
topping such as:

☐ Egg & crudités *(p.88)*
☐ Flavoured no-fat soft
   cheese *(p.42)*
☐ Red lentil & turmeric
   spread *(p.125)*
☐ Sweet potato &
   goat's cheese
   topping *(p.125)*

Lunch

Chicken or tofu reserved
from day 29 with mixed
leaf salad & tomatoes

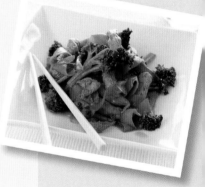

Congratulations!

You've reached the end of
The Food Doctor 30-day
Diet plan, which is great
news. I hope that you have
not only lost weight and
feel healthier, but that you
are confident about eating
healthily into the future.
Here are how some of our
Food Doctor Diet Club
members felt as they
finished the plan:

"I feel 100 per cent
confident now about
cooking healthy
meals with the right
food combinations"

Chris

"I definitely
won't be giving
up my morning
vitamin juices
and afternoon
smoothies"

Karen

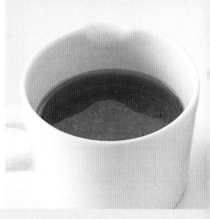

The Food Doctor

Tip for the day ...

Now that you are at the end of the 30-day Food Doctor Diet plan, read up about Principle 8, Follow the 80:20 rule *(p.137)*.

Afternoon snack

Your choice of smoothie and 1 tablespoon of mixed seeds, or Dates & fromage frais *(p.105)* or 2 oatcakes or rye biscuits, spread with a protein topping such as:

- [ ] Banana & fromage frais spread *(p.103)*
- [ ] Chick-pea & banana spread *(p.89)*
- [ ] Cottage cheese
- [ ] Classic guacamole *(p.80)*

Dinner

Fennel, carrot, broad bean & quinoa risotto with green salad *(p.164)*

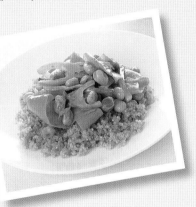

Salad dressing recipe

Store any extra dressing in a screw-top container in the fridge for up to five days.

Classic French dressing

2 tablespoons olive oil
1 teaspoon cider vinegar
1 flat teaspoon Dijon mustard
½ teaspoon red chilli paste

Mix all the ingredients together well and drizzle some dressing over a salad just before serving.

"My parents came over and it was really positive for them to see me looking so well"

Rachael

"I feel that I'm now sorted in my mind as to which foods will benefit me, and which foods won't"

Katie

"Eating the meals and snacks around a working day hasn't been an issue at all"

Brendan

Week 4 diary

Use this last week to describe how differently you feel compared to week 1 (you may like to look back to your week 1 diary and the pre-plan diary), and how confident you now feel about cooking healthy meals, combining the food groups correctly and eating well.

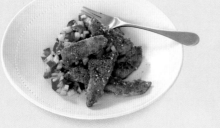

☐ DAY 24
What I've enjoyed eating/How do I feel?

- -
- -
- -
- -
- -
- -
- -
- -
- -
- -

☐ DAY 27
What I've enjoyed eating/How do I feel?

☐ DAY 28
What I've enjoyed eating/How do I feel?

☐ **DAY 25**

What I've enjoyed eating/How do I feel?

- -
- -
- -
- -
- -
- -
- -
- -
- -
- -

☐ **DAY 26**

What I've enjoyed eating/How do I feel?

- -
- -
- -
- -
- -
- -
- -
- -
- -
- -

☐ **DAY 29**

What I've enjoyed eating/How do I feel?

- -
- -
- -
- -
- -
- -
- -
- -
- -
- -

☐ **DAY 30**

What I've enjoyed eating/How do I feel?

- -
- -
- -
- -
- -
- -
- -
- -
- -
- -

Lunch ideas

Week 4 is all about starting to make your own meal choices. It's up to you which protein, vegetables and starchy carbohydrates you choose at lunchtime, so here are some suggestions.

Lunches to go

Easy proteins are a hard-boiled egg, canned tuna, smoked fish, cold chicken, seeds and chick-peas. Include a slice of rye or wholemeal bread with these lunch choices:

● 50g (2oz) sprouted seeds, ½ avocado, sliced, 1 chopped tomato, 1 tablespoon mixed seeds, 30g (1oz) feta and a dressing (pp.143,145,147).

● 50g (2oz) raw grated carrot or sweet potato, 50g (2oz) sprouted seeds tossed in a dressing of 1 tablespoon yoghurt, 1 tablespoon fromage frais, 1 tablespoon horseradish. For protein add 1 hard-boiled egg or tuna, smoked mackerel or other smoked fish.

● 4 tablespoons mixed beans or chick-peas, green leaves, raw vegetables (chopped tomatoes, cucumber, peppers, celery) and a dressing (pp.143,145,147).

● ½ can tuna with canned artichoke hearts, some mixed peppers from a jar, and a dressing (pp.143,145,147).

● If there's nothing in the house, buy your lunch from a supermarket: ready-prepared raw vegetables with some smoked fish and a dressing.

● If your supermarket has a salad bar, choose a mix of two or three salads (only one should contain pasta, couscous or rice).

● Buy some baby tomatoes and a filled wholemeal sandwich, and throw away half the bread.

Lunches at home

● Bake a small sweet potato or ordinary potato, add some mixed green leaves and 2 tablespoons of cottage cheese topped with spring onions.

● Grill sliced mushrooms and tomatoes and heat 2 tablespoons of sweet corn from a can. Mix together and pile on a slice of wholemeal toast, topped with a poached egg.

● Soften a small chopped onion in a frying pan, add a small can of chopped tomatoes, crushed garlic and chopped fresh herbs and add a can of drained and rinsed chick-peas. Simmer for 5 minutes. Add lemon juice, black pepper and ground cumin to taste.

● 75g (2½oz) prawns, 75g (2½oz) peas, ½ chopped red pepper (or use some from a jar) mixed with the juice of ½ lemon and 2 tablespoons olive oil and chopped fresh herbs. For extra flavour add a little horseradish sauce. Toast a slice of wholemeal or rye bread, drizzle with a little olive oil, pile on the prawn mix and top with some sliced spring onion.

● Make a quick stir-fry using any vegetables you have in the fridge, topped with seeds and your chosen protein (feta, tofu, cold chicken, tuna, egg, etc.). Serve with wholemeal noodles.

● Make a frittata using 2 eggs, 1 tablespoon live natural low-fat yoghurt, a small chopped onion and any fresh vegetables or peppers from a jar.

Salads

To make a healthy salad, follow these simple rules:

● 300g (10oz) vegetables per person (choose at least 5 different vegetables in a wide variety of colours)

● Mix cooked vegetables with raw (steam beans, mangetout and asparagus; red or white cabbage, broccoli, cauliflower, courgettes, grated carrot, grated sweet potato, grated celeriac, mushrooms, baby sweet corn, sprouted seeds and shelled peas are all good raw).

● Try different kinds of leaves; the paler the lettuce, the less nutrients there are.

● Sprout your own seeds for a constant supply of ultra-fresh vegetables. Put a shallow layer of seeds (alfalfa, aduki beans, etc.) in a glass jar, cover with water and cover the lid with a piece of muslin. Stand for 1 hour, then drain the water through the muslin. Rinse and drain quickly daily until the seeds have sprouted.

Stir-fries

● Use 300g (10oz) mixed vegetables per person, cut into bite-size pieces or ribbons so they cook at the same rate. If you buy a pack of ready-prepared vegetables, add some fresh vegetables too.

● Lightly blanch vegetables such as green beans and asparagus first to allow them all to cook at the same time.

● Sprouted seeds (bought or your own) add good flavour and are super-nutritious.

● Avoid olive oil; cook the vegetables in a little water or lemon juice.

● If you use seed oils, add after cooking, as the cooking process will damage them.

● Add a sauce of your choice after cooking (*p.141*).

Four ways with chicken

Use thigh fillets, which are cheaper than chicken breasts and don't dry out as much. Allow 100–150 grams (3½–5oz) of meat – approximately 2 thighs – per person. Serve with your choice of vegetables and carbohydrate. These lunch recipes serve one.

Chicken baked with tomatoes

ready in **30** minutes

1 slice wholegrain or rye bread
1x200g (7oz) can tomatoes, chopped
2 tablespoons fresh parsley, chopped
1 clove garlic, crushed
1 tablespoon lemon juice
A pinch cayenne
1 tablespoon olive oil
2 chicken thigh fillets

Preheat the oven to 180°C/350°F/gas mark 4.

Make fresh crumbs from the slice of bread (either using a coarse grater or whiz the bread in a food processor).

Combine the bread, tomatoes, parsley, garlic, lemon juice and cayenne in a saucepan, bring to the boil and simmer for a couple of minutes, stirring well.

Lightly oil an ovenproof dish with the tablespoon of oil, place the thigh fillets in the dish, pour over the sauce, cover with aluminium foil and bake for 25 minutes or so, depending on the thickness of the fillets.

Grilled chicken thighs

ready in **25** minutes

2 chicken thigh fillets
1 teaspoon olive oil

For the marinade:
1 tablespoon tamarind paste
1 tablespoon soy sauce
Juice ½ lemon
A scant tablespoon olive oil
2.5cm (1in) fresh root ginger, finely grated

Mix the marinade in a bowl and add the chicken pieces. Leave for 15 minutes (more if you have time).

Put the chicken on a lightly oiled ridged griddle over a medium-high heat, or under a medium-hot grill. Allow the chicken to brown gently, then turn the pieces over to brown the other side. Heat the remaining marinade thoroughly with a little stock, water or dry apple juice and serve as a sauce.

Stir-fried coconut chicken

ready in **30** minutes

1 tablespoon sesame seeds
1 tablespoon olive oil
1 small onion, chopped
1 clove garlic, crushed
½ green chilli chopped (optional)
2 chicken thigh fillets, cut into 5–6 thin strips
2 rounded teaspoons ground turmeric powder
1 teaspoon tamarind paste
200ml (7fl oz) coconut milk
1 small handful fresh coriander, chopped

Dry-roast the sesame seeds by putting them in a heavy pan over a medium heat for 7–8 minutes, tossing occasionally to prevent burning. Set to one side.

Heat the oil in a wok, add the onion and soften for a couple of minutes. Add the garlic, chilli and chicken pieces. Stir-fry for about 3 minutes so that the chicken browns a little. Add the turmeric, tamarind paste and 150ml (¼ pint) of the coconut milk. Simmer for about 15 minutes until the chicken is cooked. Add a little water if the sauce dries out and the chicken starts to stick.

When cooked, add the remaining coconut milk and stir. Sprinkle with sesame seeds and chopped fresh coriander.

Spicy chicken strips

ready in 30 minutes

2 chicken thigh fillets, cut into 3–4 strips
A drizzle of sesame oil

For the spicy rub:
3 teaspoons coriander seeds
6 teaspoons sesame seeds
3 teaspoons cumin seeds
½ teaspoon hot chilli

Dry-roast the coriander seeds by putting them in a heavy pan over a medium heat for 7–8 minutes, tossing occasionally to prevent burning.

Put all the spices and seeds in a grinder and whiz until ground to a powder.

Rub each strip of chicken with a little olive oil and lemon juice. Then coat each strip with the spice mix.

Cook under a medium grill or on a griddle pan for about 5 minutes on each side until cooked through, but still juicy.

Drizzle the chicken with a little sesame oil and serve with a green or red salsa (*p.165*) or 1 tablespoon live natural low-fat yoghurt and 1 tablespoon reduced-fat fromage frais mixed with lemon juice and crushed garlic.

Spicy chicken strips & salsa

Four ways with fish

Here are several options for how to cook fish, so use different varieties of fish according to your preference. Allow 100–150g (3½–5oz) of fish per person and serve with your choice of vegetables and carbohydrate. These lunch recipes serve one.

Salmon steaks with seed topping

`ready in` **25** `minutes`

3 tablespoons bought seed mix – whichever flavour you prefer – or toasted seeds *(p.51)*, zapped in a processor or grinder to make a coarse powder
¼ teaspoon ground cinnamon
2.5cm (1in) fresh ginger, grated
A little olive oil
200g (7oz) salmon steak (a little more than usual to allow for any bone in the fish)
A squeeze of lemon juice

Preheat the oven to 150°C/300°F/gas mark 2.

Mix the seed mix with the cinnamon and ginger.

Lightly oil a shallow baking dish. Place the fish fillets in the dish, squeeze over the lemon juice and season with freshly ground black pepper. Press the seed mix over the top of the fish and cover the dish with aluminium foil. Bake for about 15–20 minutes until the fish is only just cooked, and still moist. Remove the foil and slip under a hot grill for a couple of minutes to lightly brown the topping before serving.

Seared tuna with caraway seeds

`ready in` **10** `minutes`

2 teaspoons caraway seeds, crushed
¼ teaspoon cayenne pepper
100–150g (3½–5oz) tuna steak
A drizzle of olive oil
A squeeze of lemon juice

Mix the caraway seeds with the cayenne pepper and season with freshly ground black pepper. Rub the fish all over with the spices and drizzle with just a little olive oil. Cook the tuna steaks for about 3 minutes on each side on a medium-hot griddle pan (or under a medium-hot grill). The tuna should be ready when it is browning on the outside, but still moist and pink on the inside. Squeeze a little lemon juice over the fish before serving.

White fish fillets with spicy rub

`ready in` **25** `minutes`

½ teaspoon caraway seeds
½ teaspoon cumin seeds
1 teaspoon paprika
1 teaspoon cayenne
½ teaspoon black pepper
1 teaspoon dried oregano
100–150g (3½–5oz) skinless fillets of firm white fish, such as cod, haddock, hake, orange roughy or plaice
A little olive oil
A squeeze of lemon juice

Preheat the oven to 150°C/300°F/gas mark 2.

Put the caraway and cumin seeds in a grinder and whizz until finely ground to a powder. Mix the ground seeds with the remaining herbs and spices.

Rub the fish fillets with the spice mix. Lightly oil a shallow baking dish, place the fish fillets in the dish and squeeze over the lemon juice. Cover the dish with aluminium foil and bake for about 15–20 minutes, depending on the thickness of the fish. When cooked, the fish fillets should be opaque, but still moist.

Fish parcels

ready in **30** minutes

100–150g (3½–5oz) organic salmon fillets
2 tablespoons lime juice
2 teaspoons grated fresh ginger
½ teaspoon Thai fish sauce
6 good sprigs fresh fennel

Preheat the oven to 150°C/300°F/gas mark 2.

Place each fillet, skin side down, onto individual squares of aluminium foil. Fold the foil loosely into an open parcel.

Combine the lime juice, ginger and fish sauce in a bowl and pour half over each piece of fish. Top each with 2 sprigs of fennel. Seal the parcels and bake the fish for 10–15 minutes until cooked but still moist. Serve with the juice and the remaining sprigs of fennel.

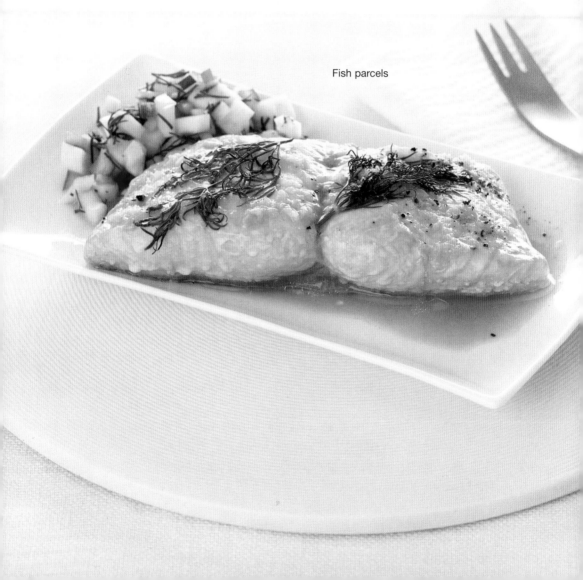

Fish parcels

Four ways with vegetarian protein

These suggestions for creating your own lunch are quick to prepare, and the ingredients are all easily available in the shops. Serve each dish with your choice of vegetables and carbohydrate. These lunch recipes all serve one.

Quinoa

ready in **15** minutes

Quinoa contains the full range of amino acids in a good balance, and therefore it makes an ideal vegetarian protein choice.

120g (4oz) quinoa
250ml (8fl oz) light stock
1 clove garlic, peeled
2 tablespoons bought fresh or The Food Doctor fresh pesto (p.84)
A squeeze of lemon juice

Simmer the quinoa in the stock with the clove of garlic. This should take about 15 minutes, by which time the stock will be absorbed and the seeds soft. Mash the garlic into the quinoa if you wish.

Stir in the fresh pesto and a good squeeze of lemon juice.

Haloumi

ready in **10** minutes

Haloumi is a firm cheese, which makes it an excellent choice for grilling or baking. It can be salty, so any sauce needs to be light.

1 tablespoon lemon juice
2.5cm (1in) fresh ginger, peeled and finely grated
1 tablespoon tamarind paste
200g (7oz) haloumi, cut in 5mm (¼in) slices

Mix the lemon juice, ginger and tamarind paste together. Place the haloumi slices on a foil-lined grill pan and brush them with the mix. Cook under a medium grill for about 4 minutes, until golden brown. Turn the slices, brush the top again and cook for a further 3–4 minutes until brown. Serve immediately, while still hot and melting.

Tofu

Although tofu is an excellent form of protein, it can taste quite bland on its own, and is best marinated in a tasty marinade for as long as possible before cooking (preferably overnight).

200g (7oz) firm tofu, cut into chunks

For the marinade:
2.5cm (1in) fresh ginger, peeled and grated
2 teaspoons Worcestershire sauce
1 teaspoon tomato purée
1 tablespoon dry apple juice
1 tablespoon balsamic vinegar
1 clove garlic, crushed

Mix the marinade and add the tofu chunks. Allow to stand for a minimum of 15 minutes. Line a grill pan with cooking foil, put the tofu pieces on top and cook under a medium grill. Turn the pieces every few minutes until they are browned on all sides.

Spicy chick-peas

ready in **10** minutes

This great source of protein can be dry fried to give the chick-peas an interesting flavour, and then added to any vegetable recipe.

1 small onion, chopped
1 tablespoon olive oil
1 tablespoon tomato purée
1 teaspoon cumin powder
¼ teaspoon chilli powder
1x400g (13oz) can chick-peas, drained and rinsed
A handful fresh coriander, chopped

Soften the onion in the olive oil in a saucepan. Add the tomato purée, cumin powder and chilli and cook together for a few seconds. Add the chick-peas and a little more olive oil if necessary. Cook over a medium-high heat until the chick-peas take on some colour. Scatter with the fresh coriander. Serve 1 portion and store the rest in the fridge for up to 5 days to use with other meals.

Spicy chick-peas with steamed vegetables

Mexican bean omelette or fritatta & salad

DINNER DAY 24

If you have any leftover bean paste, store it in the fridge to use as a spread for a morning snack. Serves two.

ready in **30** minutes

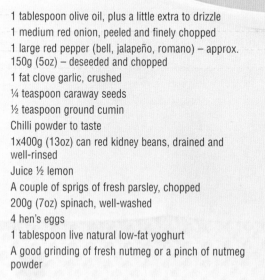

1 tablespoon olive oil, plus a little extra to drizzle
1 medium red onion, peeled and finely chopped
1 large red pepper (bell, jalapeño, romano) – approx. 150g (5oz) – deseeded and chopped
1 fat clove garlic, crushed
¼ teaspoon caraway seeds
½ teaspoon ground cumin
Chilli powder to taste
1x400g (13oz) can red kidney beans, drained and well-rinsed
Juice ½ lemon
A couple of sprigs of fresh parsley, chopped
200g (7oz) spinach, well-washed
4 hen's eggs
1 tablespoon live natural low-fat yoghurt
A good grinding of fresh nutmeg or a pinch of nutmeg powder

Heat a tablespoon of olive oil in a frying pan, add the onion and soften for about 5 minutes. Add the pepper, garlic, caraway seeds, cumin and chilli powder and season with freshly ground black pepper. Cook together for a further 5–10 minutes until the peppers are soft. Then place the mix in a food processor with the beans, lemon juice and parsley and blend to a paste. Steam the spinach until wilted and keep hot.

Beat the eggs, yoghurt and some freshly ground black pepper together. Use a non-stick omelette pan and a little oil to make two omelettes. Keep the first omelette hot while you make the second.

Put the omelettes flat on two plates, spread half the bean paste over each, top with half the spinach and a sprinkle of nutmeg. Leave flat (frittata) or fold over to make an omelette and serve with a green salad.

Fish fillet or haloumi, mushrooms & stir-fry

The mushroom topping in this recipe gives a tasty tang to your choice of fish or haloumi. Buy at least five different kinds of vegetables in a mix of colours for the stir-fry. Serves two.

60g (2½oz) chopped mushrooms (brown give a good flavour)

60g (2½oz) sundried tomatoes in olive oil, drained and chopped

A squeeze of lemon juice

200g (7oz) haloumi, sliced or 2x100–150g (3½oz–5oz) fillets of white fish (such as sole, orange roughy, cod or haddock)

A small bunch fresh parsley or coriander, chopped

For the stir-fry:

Approx. 300g (10oz) raw vegetables per person, chopped, or packet(s) of ready-prepared vegetables

Fish fillet topped with mushrooms

Combine the mushrooms, tomatoes and lemon juice. Heat a frying pan over a medium heat and gently soften the mix. Set to one side.

If using haloumi, stir-fry the vegetables first and then lightly grill the slices until golden brown, turning once. Serve topped with the mushroom mix and a good sprinkling of chopped herbs.

If using the fish fillet, preheat the oven to 180°C/350°F/gas mark 4. Lift the flesh away from the skin with a sharp knife (or ask the fishmonger to do this for you). Place each fillet on an oiled square of foil, squeeze lemon juice over each fillet and top with half the mushroom mix. Make a loose, airtight parcel of each piece of foil, place on a baking tray and bake for 15 minutes. While the fish bakes, cook the vegetables. Stir-fry them in a little water or lemon juice. If you wish, add a sauce after cooking (p.141).

Top the fish with fresh herbs and serve.

Mediterranean risotto

You can save time preparing tonight's meal by cooking the rice in advance and storing it in the fridge. Reheat the rice in a saucepan with a few tablespoons of stock. Serves two.

1 medium onion, finely sliced
1 tablespoon olive oil, plus a little to drizzle over the courgettes
100g (3½oz) red rice or brown risotto rice
200ml (7fl oz) vegetable stock
2 sprigs fresh rosemary, chopped (or 1 teaspoon dried rosemary)
2 medium courgettes, cut into 5cm (¼in) slices
1 x 250g (8oz) jar mixed roast peppers in oil
A squeeze of lemon juice
50g (2oz) feta cheese
2 lemon wedges

In a good-sized saucepan, soften the onion in the olive oil for about 5 minutes. Add the rice and stir for a few seconds. Add the stock and the rosemary, stir well and leave to simmer for about 25 minutes, or until the rice is just cooked and the stock absorbed.

Put the courgettes in a baking tray, drizzle with olive oil and toss so that the pieces are all covered with oil. Put under a medium-hot grill and brown, turning them regularly.

Drain the peppers and cut into coarse chunks.

When the rice is cooked (or reheated), mix with the vegetables and add a squeeze of lemon juice. Serve topped with a little crumbled feta cheese and a wedge of lemon to each serving.

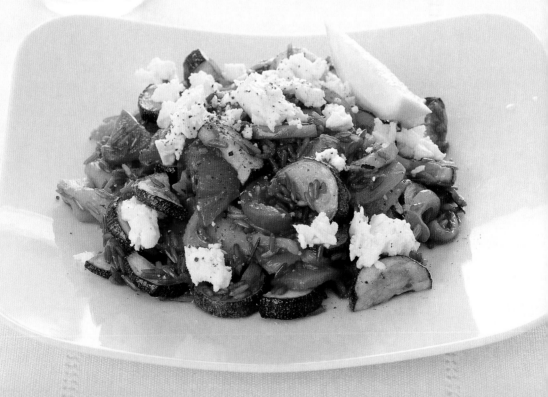

Tuscan bean soup or Mixed bean salad

Reserve a portion of soup or salad for lunch tomorrow if you wish. For extra protein in the salad, add leftover chicken or fish, feta, tofu or mixed seeds. Both recipes serve two.

Mixed bean salad

Tuscan bean soup

ready in **25** minutes

1 small onion, chopped
1 tablespoon olive oil
2 cloves garlic, peeled and chopped
2 sticks celery, sliced
1 good-sized leek, cleaned and finely sliced
1 carrot, medium, chopped
1 litre (1¾ pints) well-flavoured vegetable stock
2 bay leaves
½ teaspoon Herbes de Provence
1x400g (13oz) can mixed beans, rinsed and drained
2 tablespoons dried seaweed (optional)
1 teaspoon balsamic vinegar
1 tablespoon raw cashews, crushed

Soften the onion in a tablespoon of olive oil in a large pan. Add the garlic, celery, leek and carrot, and cook for 2 minutes. Add the stock, bay leaves and herbs. Simmer for 20 minutes. Add the beans and seaweed and simmer for 5 minutes. Stir in the vinegar and serve, sprinkled with the cashews.

Mixed bean salad

ready in **10** minutes

1x400g (13oz) can mixed beans, rinsed and drained
½ cucumber
1 large stick celery
1 carrot, medium, coarsely grated
1 red, yellow or orange bell pepper, sliced
3 medium tomatoes, quartered
Olive dressing (p.145)
2 tablespoons dried seaweed, lightly toasted under a medium grill or 2 tablespoons mixed fresh herbs, chopped

Mix the beans and fresh ingredients in the dressing. Crumble the seaweed or herbs over the top. Divide in half and serve.

Salmon or eggs with spinach & sweet potato

If you wish, save a portion of the spinach and sweet potato stir-fry, store it in the fridge and have it with your choice of protein and carbohydrate for lunch tomorrow. Serves two.

ready in 30 minutes

For the ginger topping:
2cm (¾in) cube ginger, peeled
2 small spring onions, chopped
2 sprigs dill (or 1 teaspoon dried)
Zest and juice 1 lime

2 salmon fillets (approx. 100–150g/3½–5oz each) or 2 hen's eggs
150g (5oz) sweet potato
250g (8oz) spinach leaves, washed
1 tablespoon olive oil
1 clove garlic, crushed or chopped

Salmon with spinach & sweet potato

Either prepare the ginger topping by blitzing the ingredients in a food processor, or by hand: grate the ginger, very finely chop the onions and dill, grate the lime zest, and mix together.

Preheat the oven to 160°C/320°F/gas mark 3. If using salmon, lightly oil an ovenproof dish and put in the salmon fillet skin side down. Top with the ginger mix. Cover with foil and cook for about 15 minutes, until just opaque.

If using eggs, break the eggs into 2 lightly oiled ramekin dishes. Top with the ginger mix. Bake

for about 10 minutes, or until the eggs are cooked as you like them.

Meanwhile, peel the sweet potato and cut into long ribbons using a potato peeler. Coarsely shred the spinach. Heat the oil in a frying pan or wok, add the garlic and sweet potato and gently stir-fry for about 5 minutes, until the sweet potato is hot but still crunchy. Add the spinach and cook for a further 2–3 minutes until the spinach is wilted.

Serve the vegetables topped with the salmon or eggs.

Chicken or tofu stir-fry

DINNER DAY 29

Reserve a portion of tonight's meal for lunch tomorrow if you wish. If you're short of time, use a packet of ready-prepared vegetables instead of the carrot and broccoli. Serves two.

1 tablespoon olive oil
2 chicken breasts (approx. 150g/5oz each), cut into strips, or 200g (7oz) firm tofu, cut into cubes
250g (8oz) broccoli, broken into bite-sized florets
150g (5oz) carrot, cut into matchsticks or sliced into ribbons
A drizzle of sesame oil

For the marinade:
2 tablespoons soy sauce
1 teaspoon tamarind paste
1 teaspoon five-spice paste
1 clove garlic, crushed
1 tablespoon dry apple juice
1 teaspoon cider vinegar

Mix together the marinade ingredients and leave the chicken or tofu in the marinade for a minimum of 15 minutes, and preferably as long as possible, while you prepare the vegetables.

Heat the olive oil in a wok, add the chicken or tofu pieces and brown lightly. Remove with a slotted spoon. Add the vegetables and a tablespoon of the marinade, and cook until the broccoli is just soft – the carrot will probably still be al dente. Add the chicken or tofu pieces and the rest of the marinade, bring to the boil and serve drizzled with a little sesame oil.

Chicken stir-fry

Roast vegetable quinoa & salad

DINNER DAY 30

If you can't get hold of broad beans or fennel, this recipe works well with whatever vegetables are in season. Serves two.

ready in **30** minutes

1 head fennel (150g/5oz), finely sliced lengthways

1 tablespoon olive oil

120g (4oz) quinoa

250ml (8fl oz) light vegetable stock

1 clove garlic, peeled

150g (5oz) carrot, cleaned and sliced into ribbons using a potato peeler

100g (3½oz) broad beans (weight after shelling, or use frozen)

Zest 1 orange

For the dressing:

2 tablespoons sesame oil

2 tablespoons orange juice

1 heaped teaspoon mango powder (or juice ½ lemon)

Preheat the oven to 180°C/350°F/gas mark 4. Put the fennel in a roasting pan, drizzle over the olive oil and toss well. Cook in the oven for 15 minutes or so. Meanwhile, simmer the quinoa in the stock with the garlic for about 15 minutes, or until the quinoa is just tender and the stock is absorbed. If the garlic is tender, mash it into the quinoa.

Add the carrots and broad beans to the fennel, toss well with the orange zest and season with a good grinding of black pepper. Cook for a further 10 minutes until the vegetables are cooked, but still retain some bite.

Mix the sesame oil, orange juice and mango powder or lemon juice together. Pile the quinoa onto two plates, top with the vegetables and pour over the dressing. Serve with a small mixed leaf salad.

Salsas

These salsas are a deliciously tasty addition to any meal; serve them with lunch or dinner dishes. Any leftovers can be kept in the fridge for up to three days. Each salsa serves two.

Green salsa

`ready in` **5** `minutes`

½ green pepper, very finely diced
½ small cucumber, finely diced
1 small spring onion, trimmed and finely chopped
A small handful fresh parsley, very finely chopped
1 tablespoon lemon juice
1 tablespoon olive oil
½ teaspoon soy sauce

Combine all the ingredients in a bowl. Season with some freshly ground black pepper and serve in a small side dish or bowl.

Red salsa

`ready in` **30** `minutes`

½ small red onion, finely chopped
1 medium-sized ripe tomato, skinned and chopped
½ red pepper, chopped
½ small cucumber, chopped
A couple of good sprigs of fresh basil, finely chopped (for preference, use red basil)
1 spring onion, finely chopped
1 tablespoon lime juice
1 tablespoon olive oil
1 teaspoon soy sauce

Combine all the ingredients in a bowl. Season with some freshly ground black pepper and serve in a small side dish or bowl.

If you wish, you could also zap all the ingredients together in a food processor, but take care not to process them to a purée.

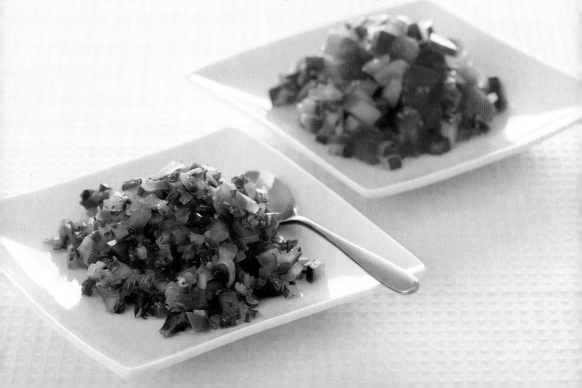

10 post-plan Diet Club members

Having completed the 30-day Food Doctor Diet plan, our Diet Club members have lost an incredible combined weight of 9 stone 5lbs (59kg). Here they describe how they felt immediately after the month was up, and how they are coping three months on.

Mary

Age 48
Height 1.73m (5ft 8½in)
New weight 79kg (12st 7lb)
Weight loss 4.5kg (10lb)
New dress size 14

As the plan became more flexible, I was aware that I needed to check I was eating the right type of food in the right proportions. By week 4 people were commenting that I looked well and slimmer, and my clothes are looser. My energy levels are now consistently better and my nails and skin have really improved; my nails usually split and tear, but for the first time in ages they are all strong and a reasonable length. I really seem to have lost the desire to binge, and I've found it easier and easier to make better food choices.

"i've lost the desire to binge"

Three months on

I've begun the first week of the plan again to kick-start me after I had a few slip-ups; I've found it relatively easy, as I know I've done it before, and it's familiar and achieveable.

Silvia

Age 39
Height 1.72m (5ft 8in)
New weight 90kg (14st 2lb)
Weight loss 5kg (11lb)
New dress size 16/18 (top/bottom)

This plan made me aware of how important it is to combine food groups correctly. Evenings are the most difficult time of the day for me. Having a young child means that I often don't get to eat my evening meal until 9pm at night, so I've followed the principles of the plan and have a snack at 4pm and again at 7pm. I'm quite confident I'll follow the main principles of The Food Doctor plan now that the month is up. They are very logical, easy to follow, and they work! I am very happy about the amount of weight I've lost. Thanks!

"I'm very happy with the weight I've lost"

Three months on
I have managed not to regain any weight, but I don't have the same energy that I had when I was following the plan. Some of the improvements have really stuck with me though: I no longer drink caffeine, I don't drink alcohol and I love having my hot lemon and ginger drink every morning.

Brendan

Age 30
Height 1.88in (6ft 2in)
New weight 90kg (14st 2lb)
Weight loss 8.2kg (18lb)
New waist size 91cm (36in)

I feel really good about the weight I've lost, as it's beyond what I'd expected. I've changed my shopping habits and buy ingredients I'd never have bought before. I'm familiar with the recipes now, and make up batches of juice and cereal quickly. I know when I need to eat and apply The Food Doctor principles; I don't ignore the signals anymore. I'm moving around a lot and spend more time on my feet. I had a blood pressure reading at the end of the plan and the results are significantly better.

"I don't ignore the signals to eat anymore"

Three months on
The 80:20 rule works for me and is beneficial to my state of mind. I feel in control of what I'm eating and find it easy to say "no" to foods that aren't going to benefit me. At the same time, I don't think I'm denying myself nice things. I've got a pretty solid routine in place now.

Rachael

Age 30
Height 1.59m (5ft 2½in)
New weight 125kg (19st 10lb)
Weight loss 9.5kg (21lb)
New dress size 24/26 (top/bottom)

My husband joined me on The Food Doctor plan and the routine has become part of our lives now. It's a great feeling. We also quickly got into a routine as a family and all sit down now to eat breakfast. It's a great time to have a good chat. I've had to make more cereals because everyone wants a taste. I've found the foods used in the plan really eye-opening, and the meals taste so good. I'm sleeping much more deeply and I'm more awake in the mornings. I'm walking wherever I can, and at a faster speed than normal. I'm continuing with the plan as I see no reason to stop.

"The routine has become part of our lives now"

Three months on

I feel so much better. I'm still drinking lots of water and eating fruit. I've not had caffeine or cola since I started the plan, which is no mean feat for me. My mum can't believe the change in my skin. I caught her staring at me, and she said she was very proud of me. I'm very proud too.

Lynne

Age 53
Height 1.70m (5ft 7in)
New weight 73kg (11st 7lb)
Weight loss 4.5kg (10lb)
New dress size 12/14 (top/bottom)

I've always eaten sensibly, but this diet has given me a better understanding of when to eat certain things and the reasons for doing so. I will keep to Ian's principle of asking, "Where's my protein?!" One thing I'll never do again is take sugar in my tea. When I had to work away from the office for four days, I made my own breakfast and lunch each day, stayed off the alcohol, went home in the evening to my Food Doctor dinner and felt great! Friends and colleagues have been really supportive and now say how well I look, which is nice. I've really enjoyed this last month and I feel great!

"Friends now say how well I look"

Three months on

I'm doing well on the 80:20 principle. I don't feel as healthy as I did while on the plan – that's because I had no alcohol for a month – but I feel so much better than I did before. I'm still caffeine-free. I've not had an indigestion tablet since day 1 of the plan and I haven't gained any of the weight I lost.

Jon

Age 36
Height 1.88m (6ft 2in)
New weight 132kg (20st 10lb)
Weight loss 7.3kg (16lb)
New waist size 123cm (48½in)

Joan

Age 32
Height 1.68m (5ft 6in)
New weight 90kg (14st 2lb)
Weight loss 5kg (11lb)
New dress size 22/18 (top/bottom)

Jon: It's been nice trying new foods such as squash, chick-peas and quinoa. I'm definitely thinking more about my food types and portion sizes. It will still take me a little more time to get to the position where I can just stick a few things together and it will meet all the requirements, but we've already gone back to recipes that we enjoyed. And I'm enjoying rooibosch (redbush) tea! I'm definitely sleeping better and I'm waking up easily. I have more energy through the day, and I seem to have a spring in my step.

Joan: I'm much more alert and have more stamina to get me through a long day. I've not had a headache for eight days – a record for me! My moods are more stable too. I've missed the occasional glass of wine, and chocolate – that's been what I've missed the most. I don't want a lot, just the odd square. I've enjoyed being part of The Food Doctor Diet club and following the plan. Thank you.

"We've already gone back to recipes that we've enjoyed"

Three months on
We found that we needed to keep a structured menu going so that we knew where we were in terms of what to eat for dinner and lunch. Because of Jon's shifts, we finally decided that we would cook for ourselves while he's on a night shift so that he can eat more sensibly. We're also hoping that we'll be able to lose a little more weight.

Katie

Age 27
Height 1.77m (5ft 10in)
New weight 79kg (12st 6lb)
Weight loss 3.2kg (7lb)
New dress size 16

I always eat breakfast, but I thought The Food Doctor breakfasts wouldn't keep me filled up. This hasn't been the case, as the breakfasts contain protein, and I've lasted until my mid-morning snack without feeling hungry. I feel that I'm now sorted in my mind as to which foods will now benefit me, and which won't. Colleagues notice that I look slimmer and healthier, and this is boosting my confidence. My skin is not as blotchy and spotty as it usually is and I'm not feeling bloated after meals. My hair looks shinier and I feel like I have lots of energy now.

"Colleagues notice that I look slimmer and healthier"

Three months on

I managed to lose some more weight and I'm now 77kg (12st 1lb). I drink only decaffeinated tea and coffee now, and have larger portions of vegetables with meals. I still look back to the recipes for ideas and inspiration – more so at weekends, when I have time to study them and do some shopping and cooking.

Chris

Age 43
Height 1.80m (5ft 11in)
New weight 86.2kg (13st 8lb)
Weight loss 5kg (11lb)
New waist size 81cm (32in)

I had really lost the pleasure of preparing meals, but I've got the cooking bug again. I'm impressed with the imaginative approach to cooking on this plan; it's also having a great effect on the way I view and respect food. Even food shopping is now fun and stimulating. I'm seeing the financial benefits of eating quality food as I'm saving a fortune on multi-vitamins. My energy levels are noticeably higher and I'm exercising more regularly. My sleep, skin and memory have improved too, so the benefits of eating healthily and exercising are clear.

"My energy levels are noticeably higher"

Three months on

I've continued to lose weight. I'm now 79.8kg (12st 8lb). I no longer need to take medication for my stomach, I have no sugar cravings and I have endless energy. I find it easy to follow the 10 principles: my new way of eating is wonderful and fulfilling.

Karen

Age 47
Height 1.70m (5ft 7in)
New weight 132kg (13st 7lb)
Weight loss 6.8kg (15lb)
New dress size 18

I am now ridiculously full of energy, and I can't remember when I last had a disturbed night's sleep. I usually have headaches at work a couple of times a week, but I don't think I've had one for over three weeks now, and I no longer have heartburn. By week 4 the plan had begun to feel less like a diet and more like a way of life. I've grown in confidence that I'll be able to keep it up now that the month is over. The proportions of my meals are much changed, and I no longer have the urge to serve every evening meal with a big plateful of rice, pasta or potatoes. I'm happy that this is the way I eat now.

"i'm happy that this is the way I eat now"

Three months on
I continued to eat healthily and lost a further 7lb (3kg). I haven't put on any of the weight I lost. I've gone from drinking a couple of cups of coffee a day before the plan to less than one a week, and I don't drink anything like as much alcohol as I used to. These are big positives for me.

Ian says

One look at these great photographs shows how well and healthy our Diet Club members seem, and how much leaner they look. I'm delighted with everyone's progress, and I'm proud of the way that they have understood and incorporated The Food Doctor plan and the 10 principles *(pp.136–37)* into their often hectic lives.

After the plan:
guidance & golden rules

If you think back to diets you've tried in the past, I wonder what happened after you finished the diet and returned to your normal way of eating? The weight probably crept back on again, leaving you at the same weight – or more – as when you started.

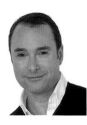

Inevitably, as we bask in the compliments that tend to come our way when we lose weight, we relax a little in the food department. You've been so good that you deserve some treats, don't you? If you gain some weight again, noone else may notice, but you do. And so you contemplate starting another diet yet again.

Changing how you eat forever

The key point here is that The Food Doctor Diet is now your normal eating pattern. It's a way of eating that means you'll never have to diet again. You will for ever more be combining protein and carbohydrates in the perfect ratio, and eating snacks in between meals each and every day, week in, week out. This will apply to your working week, your holidays, and Christmas and other celebrations throughout the year.

My 10 principles were demonstrated again and again in the plan. This pattern should have helped you to make a permanent change in the way you eat: even though the 30 days are now over, a typical week for you should still be along the lines of week 4.

Our Diet Club members

If you read the post-plan diaries of our 10 Diet Club members, you'll see that immediately after the diet everyone reported really good results. Silvia commented that my principles were very logical, and three months on she still hasn't regained any weight. Brendan reported being in a "pretty solid routine" that "feels like second nature", which is exactly what I had in mind. It's pleasing, too, that his blood pressure has come down. Katie and Chris continued to lose weight steadily, which is most encouraging. Mary repeated the first week, but I would be happier if she hadn't felt the need to repeat the first week unless it was absolutely necessary. Understanding the principles and following them consistently would have avoided the need for this. Still, I'm pleased that Mary is back on track again.

Everyone has done exceptionally well, and the reported benefits go a lot further than just weight loss. I am especially pleased that both Chris and Lynne no longer feel the need to take their stomach medication.

I hope that you are delighted with your results, and that you keep eating well and stay healthy. Just follow my 10 principles *(pp.136–37)* and my eating out tips *(right)* to continue to feel and look your very best.

Tips on eating away from home

• Before you go out for a meal or for a drink with friends, have a small snack of protein combined with carbohydrate. Feeling hungry when you order a meal invariably means you make poor food choices, while drinking on an empty stomach means the body absorbs the alcohol quickly.

• Drink plenty of water before you go out and in between each drink you order so that you minimize your alcohol consumption. If possible, drink alcohol only with a meal. Stick to red or white wine rather than spirits, beer or lager.

• Avoid foods that are almost pure carbohydrate: pizza, risotto, rice and noodles and pasta will not supply you with enough protein for your meal. And remember to avoid the bread basket.

• Desserts are a problem if you have them too often, so either apply the 80:20 rule (p.137) or use your willpower. A cheese course is better than a sugary pudding; have a small portion of cheese with a couple of crackers or a small slice of bread.

• Party snacks are also mostly simple carbohydrates. Avoid savoury crackers and crisps and have a few raw, unsalted nuts or some olives instead.

• If you are eating out with kids, don't be tempted to eat in their favourite fast-food restaurant, or pick at their plates of food. Find a restaurant with a varied, healthy menu that you can all enjoy. Choose lean proteins for yourself, such as tuna or chicken, and some vegetables.

• If a friend or your family invites you round for a meal, the answer lies in which foods you leave out rather than what you replace them with. Make sure you ask for a large serving of vegetables and a small serving of carbohydrate if it's lunchtime; if you're eating dinner, leave out the starchy carbohydrates altogether.

• Don't lose weight before a holiday, only to put it back on again while you're away. Stick to The Food Doctor principles and you should be fine. You can rip out pp.179-80 and bring them

with you on holiday to remind yourself of the principles. You should also limit your alcohol intake during the day and have a small snack before you eat dinner so that you don't feel tempted to choose unsuitable dishes.

• Always keep some fruit – preferably hard fruit such as apples or pears – and a supply of raw, unsalted nuts to hand for snacks while you are travelling or on holiday, but don't eat the nuts all at once: six or seven nuts will be enough with one piece of fruit.

• If you are travelling and have to buy yourself a meal, include enough lean protein. If you buy a sandwich, discard half the bread to make one generously filled sandwich. If you're travelling with children, fill a plastic container with sliced raw vegetables, grapes, cherry tomatoes and pieces of hard cheese to help them – and you – avoid fast-food snacks and meals.

Tapenade fish fillet or Tapenade tofu

The fish or the tofu both go well with Warm lentil salad *(p.61)*, or serve either with roasted cherry tomatoes and a green leaf salad or a vegetable stir-fry. Serves two.

Tapenade fish fillet

ready in **10** minutes

1 good tablespoon tapenade
2 teaspoons lemon juice
150g (5oz) firm white fish fillets
(cod, haddock, monkfish, etc.)
1 scant tablespoon
olive oil

Tapenade
fish fillet

Mix the tapenade and lemon juice

If using fish, cut the fish fillets into strips approximately 2cm (¾in) wide. Allow them to steep in the tapenade mixture for a few minutes.

Heat the olive oil in a frying pan, and over a gentle heat add the fish. Cook each side for a couple of minutes. Serve immediately.

Tapenade tofu

ready in **5** minutes

2 tablespoons tapenade
2–3 tablespoons lemon juice
150g (5oz) tofu, sliced

Mix the tapenade with the lemon juice. Brush the tofu with the tapenade mix and grill, turning once, until lightly brown and crispy. Serve immediately.

Carrot & cardamom stuffed squash

If you have the time to prepare this meal, it makes for a wonderful tasty and colourful dish. A quicker version that omits the gem squashes is on page 98. Serves two.

50g (2oz) red or brown rice
250ml (8fl oz) vegetable stock
2 tablespoons dried sea vegetables or spinach
2 hen's eggs
1 tablespoon olive oil, plus a little extra for scrambling the eggs
2 gem squashes, or similar-sized squashes in season
5 cardamom pods
1 small onion, chopped
100g (3½oz) carrot, coarsely grated
Zest 1 orange, grated

Simmer the rice in the stock for 25 minutes or so, until just tender. Add the dried sea vegetables or spinach and stir for a couple of minutes. If there is any liquid left, turn up the heat and boil until the liquid is absorbed. Set aside.

In a non-stick pan, scramble the two eggs in just a little oil. Set aside.

Cut each gem squash in half, scrape out the seeds and put each half in a steamer. Steam for about 10 minutes until the flesh is beginning to soften, but not thoroughly cooked.

Make a slit in each cardamom pod, scrape the seeds into a pestle and crush with a mortar. Heat the oil in a frying pan and soften the onion for a few minutes. Add the crushed seeds and stir, then add the grated carrot and orange zest. Cook for about 5 minutes until the carrot softens. Stir in the cooked rice and fold in the scrambled egg.

Pile the mix into the squashes, place in a shallow baking dish, cover and cook for about 15 minutes in a hot oven. Serve with a green leaf salad.

Turkey escalopes

This is a quick and easy way to cook turkey, or even chicken if you prefer. Serve the escalopes with a variety of steamed vegetables and your choice of salsa (p.165). Serves two.

ready in **20** minutes

2 escalopes of turkey (approx 100g/3½oz each)
1 clove garlic, crushed
Juice 1 lemon
1 tablespoon olive oil

If the escalopes are not paper thin, put each piece of meat between two sheets of greaseproof paper and beat them flat with a rolling pin. Lay the escalopes in a shallow dish and rub in the garlic. Sprinkle with lemon juice and season with a good grinding of fresh black pepper. Leave to marinade for a minimum of 15 minutes.

Heat the olive oil in a frying pan or wok over a medium-high heat. Lift the escalopes from the marinade and brown each side in the pan – this should take about 2 minutes. Place each escalope on a plate and serve with steamed vegetables and a salsa of your choice.

Mixed vegetable rosti

DINNER

Choose a variety of colours and dark green vegetables for this rosti; the only essential item is a small onion. Serves two.

ready in **30** minutes

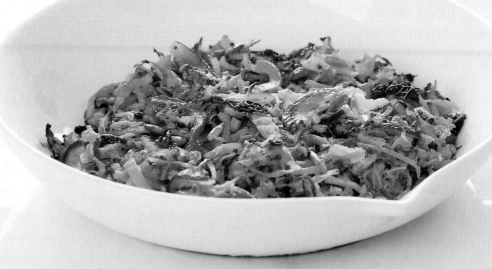

600g (1lb 4oz) mixed vegetables (choose about half as root vegetables: sweet potato, celeriac, carrot, parsnip, turnip, onion, leek – including the green parts, and so on; the remainder can be peppers of any colour, squash, courgettes, kale, green cabbage, spinach, etc.)

3 tablespoons olive oil

1 tablespoon black mustard seeds

2 tablespoons sesame seeds or mixed seeds *(p.51)*

2 cloves garlic, crushed

Clean and grate or finely shred the vegetables (wash any leeks thoroughly after shredding).

Heat 2 tablespoons of olive oil in a small pan, add the black mustard seeds, and swirl round over the heat until the seeds start to pop. Put the popped mustard seeds and the sesame or mixed seeds in a large bowl and add the vegetables and garlic. Season with freshly ground black pepper and mix the ingredients all together.

Heat a scant tablespoon of olive oil in a non-stick frying pan (use a little more oil if the pan is not non-stick). Add the vegetables and cook for about 10 minutes, stirring occasionally, until they are soft. Press the mixture evenly over the pan to form a "cake" and leave to brown a little on the bottom for about 5 minutes. Then slip the pan under a medium-hot grill to brown the top.

This rosti could be served with different sources of protein: baked trout *(p.92)*, grilled haloumi *(p.156)*, feta cheese, poached egg, or baked chicken or turkey fillets.

Coconut stir-fry

DINNER

This tasty stir-fry goes very well with Salmon cakes or Egg noodles *(p.122),* or choose your own protein to serve with it. Serves two.

ready in **10** minutes

1 tablespoon olive oil

50g (2oz) mangetout or green beans, topped and tailed

50g (2oz) red pepper, cut into strips

50g (2oz) yellow pepper, cut into strips

50g (2oz) red onion, finely sliced

100g (3½oz) carrot or sweet potato, cut into ribbons using a potato peeler

150ml (½ pint) coconut milk (or use 50g/2oz of creamed coconut dissolved in 100ml/3½fl oz hot water)

Juice ½ lime

A small handful fresh coriander or basil leaves, chopped

Heat the olive oil in a wok, add all the vegetables and cook together for about 5 minutes, until the vegetables are all cooked al dente (the mangetout or beans will take the longest). Stir in the coconut milk and lime juice and season with freshly ground black pepper. Serve the stir-fry topped with the fresh herbs and your choice of protein.

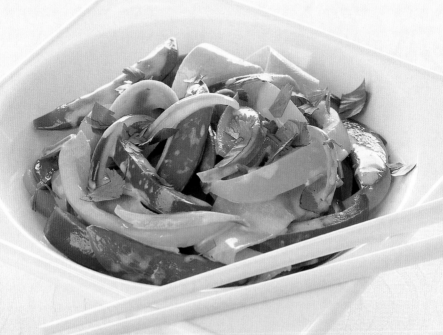

10 Principles

1 Eat protein with complex carbohydrates

Combining these food groups in the right proportions will give you a steady flow of energy, as the body converts foods relatively slowly into glucose. You can then avoid triggering insulin production, therefore minimizing the potential for your body to store food as fat.

2 Stay hydrated

Drink at least 1.5 litres (3½ pints) of water a day, and more in hot weather or if you are exercising. Remember, by the time you feel thirsty you are already dehydrated. Limit your alcohol and salt intake too, as they dehydrate the body.

3 Eat a wide variety of food

Avoid getting stuck in a routine when shopping. Most of us buy the same 10 per cent of foods for 90 per cent of the time. Try to buy two new foods every week.

4 Fuel up frequently

Eat the right foods little and often. This gives you a constant supply of energy, avoiding insulin production, hunger, tiredness and food cravings. So although you eat more regularly at set times of the day, you still lose weight.

5 Eat breakfast

A balanced breakfast supplies the fuel to help maintain energy levels and set your metabolism up for the day. Eating breakfast is fundamental to controlling your weight and feeling energetic in the long term.

6 Avoid sugar

Sugar breaks down into glucose extremely quickly, therefore contributing to fat production and weight gain. This creates a high, and the resulting low causes hunger. Avoiding sugar also helps you achieve good digestive health.

7 Exercise is essential

Healthy eating must go hand-in-hand with exercise. Exercise increases your metabolic rate – the speed at which your body uses up food as energy. Aim to fit in 30 minutes of exercise three times a week.

8 Follow the 80:20 rule

It is perfectly normal to stray every now and then. If you follow The Food Doctor principles and meal plan for 80 per cent of the time, you can stray for 20 per cent without feeling guilty. This means you can enjoy social occasions and also escape the boredom and frustration that is associated with diet regimes.

9 Make time to eat

Try not to eat in a hurry and chew each mouthful thoroughly. Taking time over a meal is beneficial to digestive health. Your food will also taste more satisfying.

10 Eat fat to lose fat

Fat is not always the enemy. The body needs certain essential fats (omega-3 and omega-6) to function properly. It is saturated fat that you need to avoid. Aim to include essential fats in your diet up to four or five times a week.

Tips on eating away from home

● Before you go out for a drink with friends or a meal, have a small snack of protein combined with carbohydrate. Feeling hungry when you order a meal invariably means you make poor food choices, while drinking on an empty stomach means the body absorbs the alcohol quickly. Have the confidence to order to eat in a way that suits you.

● Drink plenty of water before you go out and in between drinks to minimize your alcohol consumption. If possible, drink alcohol only with a meal. Stick to red or white wine rather than spirits, beer or lager.

● Avoid foods that are almost pure carbohydrate: pizza, risotto, rice and noodles and pasta will not supply you with enough protein for your meal. And avoid the bread basket.

● Desserts are a problem if you have them too often, so you either need to apply the 80:20 rule (p.179), or use your willpower. A cheese course is better than a sugary pudding, but make sure you have a small portion of cheese.

● Party snacks are also mostly simple carbohydrates. Avoid savoury crackers and crisps and have a few raw, unsalted nuts or olives instead.

● If you are eating out with kids, don't be tempted to eat in their favourite fast-food restaurant, or pick at their food. Find a restaurant with a varied, healthy menu that you can all enjoy. Choose lean proteins for yourself, such as tuna or chicken, and some vegetables.

● If a friend or your family invites you round for a meal, the situation can create problems, as you're not in control of what you're eating. There's no need to offend anyone and avoid the meal altogether: the answer lies in which foods you leave out rather than what you replace them with. Make sure you ask for a large serving of vegetables and a small serving of carbohydrate if it's lunchtime; if you're eating dinner, leave out the carbohydrates altogether.

● Don't lose weight before a holiday, only to put it back on again while you're away. Stick to The Food Doctor principles and you should be fine. For example, avoid continental breakfasts and order a breakfast that includes enough protein. You won't use up much energy if you're lying on the beach or by the pool, so don't eat large, carbohydrate-laden lunches. Limit your alcohol intake during the day and have a small snack before you eat dinner.

● Keep some fruit – preferably hard fruit such as apples or pears – and a supply of raw, unsalted nuts to hand for snacks while you are travelling or on holiday, but don't eat the nuts all at once: eight or nine nuts will be enough with one piece of fruit.

● If you are travelling and have to buy yourself a meal, make sure your meal includes enough lean protein. If you buy a sandwich, discard half the bread to make one generously filled sandwich. In this way you'll have a more favourable ratio of protein to carbohydrates. If you're travelling with children, fill a plastic container with sliced raw vegetables, grapes, cherry tomatoes and pieces of hard cheese to help them – and you – avoid fast-food snacks and meals.

Shopping list: Prep days & soups

☐ Apples, 4

☐ Bananas, 1

☐ Lemons, 2

☐ Limes, 1

☐ Pears, 1

☐ Carrots, approx. 50g (2oz)

☐ Cherry tomatoes, 1 tub

☐ Cucumbers, small, 2

☐ Mixed raw vegetables, approx. 600g (1lb 3½oz)

☐ Mixed salad ingredients: enough for 2 portions

☐ Onions, medium, 1

☐ Onions, small, 2

☐ Peppers, green, 1

☐ Peppers, red, 1

☐ Red onion, small, 1

☐ Spring onions, 1 bunch

☐ Sweet potatoes, large, 1

☐ Tomatoes, medium, 2

☐ Basil, fresh, 1 packet

☐ Parsley, fresh, 1 bunch

☐ Hen's eggs, 1

☐ Live natural low-fat yoghurt, 1 large pot

☐ Haloumi, 200g (7oz) (if making Oat-crumb haloumi, day 2)

☐ Beef mince, very lean, 200g (7oz) (if making Beef burgers, day 1)

☐ White fish fillet , 200g (7oz), (if making Oat-crumb fish, day 2)

☐ Orange or apple juice, 1 carton

☐ Peppermint tea, 1 packet

☐ *Chick-peas, 1x400g (13oz) can (if making Chick-pea burgers, day 1)

☐ Oatcakes, 1 packet

☐ Oat flakes, 1 packet

☐ Rice, Camargue (red) or brown, 1 packet

☐ Mixed seeds, 1 tub

☐ Nuts, raw unsalted, 1 small packet

☐ Chilli powder, 1 jar

☐ Cumin powder, 1 small jar

☐ Herbes de Provence (dried), 1 pot

☐ Mustard, 1 small pot

☐ Olive oil, 1 large bottle

☐ Soy sauce, 1 bottle

☐ Stock, light vegetable, 150ml (¼ pint) OR yeast-free bouillon powder, 1 tub

FOR THE WINTER SOUPS

☐ Carrots, 500g (1lb 2oz)

☐ Celery, 1 bunch

☐ Garlic bulbs, 1

☐ Leeks, medium, 1

☐ Onions, medium, 1

☐ Onions, small, 1

☐ Red pepper, large, 1

☐ Watercress, fresh, 2 bunches

☐ *Cannellini beans, 1x400g (13oz) can

☐ *Chick-peas, 1x400g (13oz) can

☐ Plum tomatoes, chopped, 1x400g (13oz) can

☐ Basil (dried), 1 small jar

☐ Mango powder, 1 jar

☐ Smoked paprika, 1 small jar

☐ Vegetable stock, 2 litres (3½ pints) OR yeast-free bouillon powder, 1 tub

FOR THE SUMMER SOUPS

☐ Lemons, 2

☐ Baby corn, 100g (3½oz)

☐ Carrots, 100g (3½oz)

☐ Cucumber, ½

☐ Baby leeks 100g (3½oz) OR spring onions, 1 bunch

☐ Mangetout, 100g (3½oz)

☐ Pepper, 1 (any colour)

☐ Red onion, medium, 1

☐ Coriander, fresh, 1 bunch

☐ Ginger, fresh root, 1 piece

☐ Apple juice, 1 carton

☐ Vegetable juice, 1 carton

☐ *Cannellini beans, 1x400g (13oz) can

☐ Plum tomatoes, chopped, 1x400g (13oz) can

☐ Quinoa, 1 packet

☐ Miso paste, 1 packet

☐ Tomato purée, 1 tube

☐ Tabasco, 1 bottle

☐ Vegetable stock, 1.6 litres (2¾ pints) OR yeast-free bouillon powder, 1 tub

*All cans should be free from added salt and sugar

Shopping list: storecupboard food

- [ ] Barley flakes, 1 packet
- [ ] Buckwheat flour, 1 packet
- [ ] Quinoa flakes, 1 packet
- [ ] Quinoa seeds, 1 packet
- [ ] Rice, wholegrain puffed, 1 packet
- [ ] Oatcakes, approx. 4 packets
- [ ] Rye biscuits, approx. 2 packets
- [ ] Corn pasta shells, 1 packet
- [ ] Quinoa, 1 packet
- [ ] Lentils, dried puy, 1 packet
- [ ] Lentils, red, 1 packet
- [ ] Dried sea vegetables (optional) 1–2 packets
- [ ] Dried seaweed, 1 packet
- [ ] Mixed seeds, 1 tub (if not already bought for prep days) OR 1 packet each sunflower, sesame, pumpkin & linseeds
- [ ] Sesame seeds, 1 small packet
- [ ] Sunflower seeds, 1 small packet
- [ ] Cashew nuts, raw unsalted, 1 packet
- [ ] Mixed nuts, raw unsalted, 1 packet
- [ ] Herb teas, 1–2 packets (e.g. peppermint, lemon rooibosch, camomile)
- [ ] Apricots, dried, 1 packet

- [ ] Raisins, 1 small packet
- [ ] Balsamic vinegar, 1 bottle
- [ ] Cider vinegar, 1 bottle
- [ ] Olive oil, 1 bottle (if not already bought for prep days and soups)
- [ ] Sesame oil, 1 bottle
- [ ] Soy sauce, 1 bottle (if not already bought for prep days and soups)
- [ ] *Butter beans, 1x400g (13oz) can
- [ ] *Cannellini beans, 1x400g (13oz) can
- [ ] *Chick-peas, approx. 5x400g (13oz) cans
- [ ] Coconut milk, 1x400g (13oz) can (or 50g/2oz creamed coconut)
- [ ] *Lentils, 1x400g (13oz) can
- [ ] *Mixed beans, 1x400g (13oz) can
- [ ] Passata, 1x500ml (17fl oz) carton
- [ ] *Puy lentils, 1x400g (13oz) can
- [ ] Plum tomatoes, approx. 2x400g (13oz) cans
- [ ] *Red kidney beans, 1x400g (13oz) can
- [ ] Black olives, 1 jar
- [ ] Dijon mustard, 1 pot
- [ ] Five-spice paste, 1 jar (also called Chinese five-spice paste)
- [ ] Five-spice powder, 1 jar (also called Chinese

- five-spice powder)
- [ ] Hot horseradish sauce, 1 jar
- [ ] Mixed roast peppers, 1 jar
- [ ] Sun-dried tomatoes, 1 jar
- [ ] Tamarind paste, 1 jar
- [ ] Tabasco sauce (or cayenne pepper), 1 bottle
- [ ] Tapenade, 1 jar
- [ ] Thai fish sauce, 1 bottle
- [ ] Worcestershire sauce, 1 bottle
- [ ] Black peppercorns, 1 packet
- [ ] Black mustard seeds, 1 packet
- [ ] Caraway (or fennel) seeds, 1 packet
- [ ] Cardamom pods, 1 jar
- [ ] Cayenne pepper, 1 jar
- [ ] Celery seeds, 1 packet
- [ ] Cinnamon powder, 1 jar
- [ ] Cinnamon stick, 1
- [ ] Curry powder, 1 jar
- [ ] Dried dill, 1 jar
- [ ] Mixed dried herbs, 1 jar
- [ ] Nutmeg (fresh or dried)
- [ ] Turmeric powder, 1 jar
- [ ] Yeast-free bouillon powder, 1 tub (if not already bought for soups and prep days)

*All cans should be free from added salt and sugar

Shopping list: week 1

FRESH FOOD FOR DAYS 3–9

This shopping list includes approximate quantities for all meals and snacks in Week 1. You may need to replace some items during the week.

- [ ] Apples, approx. 3
- [ ] Berries, fresh or frozen, approx. 600g (1lb 3½oz)
- [ ] Lemons, approx. 12
- [ ] Limes, 1
- [ ] Oranges, 6
- [ ] Pears, approx. 7
- [ ] Pomegranate, 1 (optional)
- [ ] Asparagus spears, 12 (or 2 plump heads of red or green chicory)
- [ ] Butternut or acorn squash, 1 (or choose any other firm-fleshed squash)
- [ ] Carrots, small, 1
- [ ] Courgettes, medium, 1
- [ ] Garlic, 1 bulb
- [ ] Mangetout, 150g (5oz)
- [ ] Mixed raw vegetables, approx. 500g (1lb) or equivalent weight of ready-prepared vegetables in packets
- [ ] Mixed salad ingredients: enough for 6 portions
- [ ] Onions, small, 3
- [ ] Pepper (yellow or green), 1
- [ ] Red onion, medium, 1

- [ ] Red peppers (romano if possible), 2
- [ ] Rocket leaves (optional), 1 packet
- [ ] Shallots, 3
- [ ] Spring onions, 1 bunch
- [ ] Sprouted seeds (if not growing your own), 1 tub
- [ ] Tomatoes, medium-large, 3 (or 1x200g/7oz can chopped tomatoes)
- [ ] Watercress, fresh, 1 bunch
- [ ] Basil, fresh, 1 bunch
- [ ] Coriander, fresh, 1 bunch
- [ ] Ginger, fresh root, 1 large-sized piece
- [ ] Parsley, fresh, 1 bunch
- [ ] Sage, fresh, 1 bunch
- [ ] Cottage cheese (optional), 1 large tub
- [ ] Feta cheese, 1 packet
- [ ] Haloumi, 1 packet (if using on day 5)
- [ ] Hen's eggs, 11
- [ ] Live natural low-fat yoghurt, 1 large pot
- [ ] Milk, whole or semi-skimmed, 1 pint
- [ ] No-fat soft cheese, 1 large tub
- [ ] Parma ham (or good-quality ham), 4 thin slices (if using on day 5)
- [ ] Reduced-fat fromage frais, 1 tub

- [ ] Tofu, 200g (7oz) (if making Spicy tofu, day 7)
- [ ] Rye bread, 1 loaf
- [ ] Wholemeal bread, 1 loaf
- [ ] Apple juice, dry or unsweetened, 1 carton
- [ ] Carrot juice, fresh, 725ml (1¼ pints)
- [ ] Mixed vegetable juice, 725ml (1¼ pints)
- [ ] Nut or soya milk, approx 550ml (19fl oz)
- [ ] Chicken joints (leg and thigh), 2 (if making Spicy chicken, day 7)
- [ ] Tuna steaks, 2, approx. 100g (3½oz) each (if making Tuna in spicy tomato sauce, day 4)
- [ ] Plum tomatoes, 1x200g (7oz) can (if making Tuna in spicy tomato sauce, day 4)
- [ ] Light vegetable stock, 1.2 litres (2 pints)

Note:

If you need to buy suitable plastic containers to transport your food, buy two containers for your lunches and snacks, and two for your morning and afternoon drinks

Shopping list: week 2

FRESH FOOD FOR DAYS 10–16

This shopping list includes approximate quantities for seven supper recipes and five weekday lunches. It does not include ingredients for your choice of breakfasts, snacks, or weekend brunches or lunches.

- [ ] Lemons, 2
- [ ] Limes, approx. 3
- [ ] Oranges, 2
- [ ] Asparagus, 100g (3½oz)
- [ ] Avocado, 1
- [ ] Beetroot, raw or ready-cooked, 150g (5oz)
- [ ] Carrots, medium, 2
- [ ] Cherry tomatoes, 1 large tub
- [ ] Chicory, medium, 2 (or 2 gem lettuce)
- [ ] Courgettes, medium, 1
- [ ] Fennel, medium, 1
- [ ] Mixed green vegetables (eg, French beans, runner beans, mangetout, asparagus), approx. 450g (15oz)
- [ ] Mixed raw vegetables, approx. 600g (1lb 3½oz) or equivalent weight of ready-prepared vegetables in packets
- [ ] Mixed salad ingredients: enough for 9 portions
- [ ] Mushrooms, small, 150g (5oz), plus 8
- [ ] mushrooms (if making Vegetable brochettes, day 12)
- [ ] Onions, small, 4
- [ ] Onions, medium, 2
- [ ] Peppers, red, 3
- [ ] Peppers, yellow, 2
- [ ] Spinach (fresh or frozen) or kale, 100g (3½oz)
- [ ] Sprouted seeds (if not growing your own), 1 tub
- [ ] Coriander, fresh, 1 bunch
- [ ] Ginger, fresh root, 1 large piece
- [ ] Parsley, fresh, 1 bunch
- [ ] Feta cheese, 150g (5oz)
- [ ] Haloumi, 200g (7oz) (if making Grilled haloumi, day 10)
- [ ] Hen's eggs, 3
- [ ] Reduced-fat fromage frais, 1 tub
- [ ] Tofu, 200–250g (7–8oz) (if making Smoked tofu salad, day 14)
- [ ] Dry apple juice, 1 carton
- [ ] Chicken thigh fillets, 250–300g (8–11oz) (if making Chicken brochettes, day 12)
- [ ] Duck breasts, 2, approx. 200g (7oz) each (if making Duck breast salad, day 14)
- [ ] Trout, 2, approx. 200g (7oz) after removing the head and tail (if making Baked trout, day 10)
- [ ] Tuna, 1 small can for lunch, day 10, and 1 large can (if you have run out) for lunch, day 16
- [ ] Rye biscuits or rice cakes, 1 packet (if you have run out)

DAY 13 DINNER OPTIONS

Quick country soup

- [ ] Lemons, 1
- [ ] Mushrooms, button, 400g (13oz)
- [ ] Onions, medium, 1
- [ ] Dried sea vegetables, 1 small packet, or spinach, 50g (2oz)
- [ ] Vegetable stock, 500ml (17fl oz)

Four bean salad

- [ ] Lemons, 1
- [ ] Broad beans, 100g (3½oz)
- [ ] Green beans, 100g (3½oz)
- [ ] Mangetout or petit pois, 100g (3½oz)
- [ ] Onion, medium, 1
- [ ] Pepper, 1 (red or orange)
- [ ] Spring onions, 1 bunch
- [ ] Fresh herbs of your choice, 1 bunch
- [ ] Feta cheese, 50g (optional)
- [ ] Cannellini beans, 1x400g (13oz) can (if you have run out)

Shopping list: week 3

FRESH FOOD FOR DAYS 17–23

This shopping list includes approximate quantities for seven supper recipes and five weekday lunches. It does not include ingredients for your choice of breakfasts, snacks, or weekend brunches or lunches.

- [ ] Lemons, approx. 4
- [ ] Limes, 2
- [ ] Aubergines, 1 (approx. 200g/7oz)
- [ ] Beefsteak tomatoes, 2
- [ ] Carrots, small, 1 (if making Vegetarian burgers, day 23)
- [ ] Cherry tomatoes, 1 tub
- [ ] Courgettes, 500g (1lb)
- [ ] Mixed salad ingredients: enough for 9 portions
- [ ] Mixed raw vegetables, approx. 850g (approx. 2lb) or equivalent weight of ready-prepared vegetables in packets
- [ ] Mushrooms, large, 4
- [ ] Onions, medium, 1
- [ ] Shiitake mushrooms, 4 (if making Vegetarian burgers, day 23)
- [ ] Spring onions, 1 bunch
- [ ] Sprouted seeds, 1 tub (if you are not growing your own)
- [ ] Sweet potatoes, medium, 1

- [ ] Tomatoes, large, 5
- [ ] Coriander, fresh, 1 packet
- [ ] Ginger, fresh root, 1 large piece (if you have run out)
- [ ] Parsley, fresh, 1 bunch
- [ ] Black olives, 8–10
- [ ] Cottage cheese, 1 tub
- [ ] Feta or haloumi cheese, 200g (7oz) (if using cheese, day 22)
- [ ] Hen's eggs, 4 (3 if making Egg noodles, day 21, 1 if making Vegetarian burgers, day 23)
- [ ] Live natural low-fat yoghurt, 1 large pot (if you have run out)
- [ ] Smoked tofu, 100g (3½oz) if making Stir-fry tofu, day 19
- [ ] Tofu, 200g (7oz) (if making Vegetarian burgers, day 23)
- [ ] Rye bread, 1 loaf
- [ ] Chicken, 100g (3½oz) (if making Stir-fry chicken, day 19)
- [ ] Chicken or turkey, minced, 300g (10oz) (if making Chicken burgers, day 23)
- [ ] Salmon fillet, 150–200g (5–7oz) (if making Salmon cakes, day 21)
- [ ] White fish fillet, 250–300g (8–10oz) (if using fish, day 22)

DAY 20 DINNER OPTIONS
Salade niçoise

- [ ] Carrot, medium, 1
- [ ] Gem lettuce or similar, 1
- [ ] Green or runner beans, 100g (3½oz)
- [ ] Pepper, yellow, 1
- [ ] Spring onions, 1 bunch
- [ ] Tomatoes, medium, 2
- [ ] Fresh herbs of your choice, 1 bunch
- [ ] Hen's eggs 1 (2 if making vegetarian option)
- [ ] Black olives, 6–8
- [ ] Tuna steak, fresh, 1 or 1 large can of tuna in spring water (if making traditional salad niçoise)
- [ ] Chick-peas, 1x400g (13oz) can (if you have run out and are making Spicy chick-peas)

Leek & potato soup

- [ ] Leeks, large, 1
- [ ] Onions, medium, 1
- [ ] Sweet potato, medium, 1
- [ ] Dried sea vegetables, 1 small packet
- [ ] Quinoa, 100g (3½oz) (if you have run out)
- [ ] Light vegetable stock 250ml (8fl oz)

Shopping list: week 4

This shopping list includes approximate quantities for seven supper recipes only. It does not include ingredients for your choice of breakfasts, snacks, brunches or lunches.

- [ ] Lemons, approx. 3
- [ ] Limes, 1
- [ ] Oranges, 1
- [ ] Broad beans, 100g (3½oz)
- [ ] Broccoli, 250g (8oz)
- [ ] Carrots, approx. 300g (10oz)
- [ ] Courgettes, medium, 2
- [ ] Fennel, 1
- [ ] Mixed raw vegetables, approx. 600g (1lb 3½oz) or equivalent weight of ready-prepared vegetables in packets
- [ ] Mixed salad ingredients: enough for 4 portions
- [ ] Mushrooms (brown), 60g (2½oz)
- [ ] Onions, medium, 1
- [ ] Peppers, red (bell, jalopeno or romano), large, 1, OR 1 jar red peppers
- [ ] Red onions, medium, 1
- [ ] Spinach, fresh, 450g (15oz)
- [ ] Spring onions, 1 bunch
- [ ] Sweet potatoes, medium, 1
- [ ] Tomatoes, medium, 1
- [ ] Coriander, fresh, 1 bunch

- [ ] Dill, fresh, 1 bunch
- [ ] Fresh ginger, 1 large piece (if you have run out)
- [ ] Garlic, 1 bulb (if you have run out)
- [ ] Parsley, fresh, 1 bunch
- [ ] Rosemary, fresh, 1 bunch
- [ ] Feta cheese, 1 packet
- [ ] Haloumi, 1 packet (if making Haloumi & mushrooms, day 25)
- [ ] Hen's eggs, 4 (plus 2 if making Ginger eggs, day 28)
- [ ] Live natural low-fat yoghurt, 1 large pot (if you have run out)
- [ ] Tofu, 1 packet (if making Tofu stir-fry, day 29)
- [ ] Chicken breasts, approx. 300g (10oz) (if making Chicken stir-fry, day 29)
- [ ] Salmon fillets, 2, approx. 200–300g (7–10oz) (if making Ginger salmon, day 28)
- [ ] White fish fillets (sole, orange roughy, cod, haddock), 200–300g (7–10oz) (if making Fish & mushrooms, day 25)
- [ ] Mixed roast peppers in oil, 250g (8oz) jar, 1
- [ ] Sundried tomatoes, 60g (2½oz)
- [ ] Dry apple juice, 1 carton
- [ ] Camargue (red) or brown risotto rice, 1

- [ ] packet (if you have run out)
- [ ] Red kidney beans, 1x400g (13oz) can (if you have run out)
- [ ] Vegetable stock, 550ml (19fl oz)

DAY 27 DINNER OPTIONS

Tuscan bean soup

- [ ] Carrots, medium, 1
- [ ] Celery, 2 sticks
- [ ] Leeks, large, 1
- [ ] Onions, small, 1
- [ ] Mixed beans, 1x400g (13oz) can
- [ ] Dried sea vegetables, 1 small packet (optional)
- [ ] Raw cashews, 1 small packet (if you have run out)
- [ ] Vegetable stock, 1 litre (1¾ pints)

Mixed bean salad

- [ ] Carrot, medium, 1
- [ ] Celery, 1 stick
- [ ] Cucumber, ½
- [ ] Pepper (red/yellow/orange), 1
- [ ] Tomatoes, medium, 3
- [ ] Mixed beans, 1x400g (13oz) can
- [ ] Dried sea vegetables or seaweed, 1 small packet

Index

About the author

Ian Marber

MBANT Dip ION

Nutrition consultant, author, broadcaster
and health journalist

Ian studied at the Institute for Optimum Nutrition, and now heads The Food Doctor clinic at Notting Hill, London. He contributes regularly to many of Britain's leading magazines and newspapers and appears regularly on TV and radio shows. He has also made a 15-part series for the Discovery Health channel. He is currently studying for a master's degree in nutrition therapy.

Undiagnosed food sensitivities in his twenties led to Ian becoming interested in nutrition. His condition was later identified as coeliac disease, a life-long intolerance to gluten. He is now an acknowledged expert on nutrition and digestion, and many of his clients are referred to his clinic by doctors and gastroenterologists.

Ian advises on all aspects of nutrition, in particular on the impact that correct food choices can have on health. He is known to give motivational, positive and practical advice that can make a real difference to your well-being.

Ian's first book, *The Food Doctor – Healing Foods for Mind and Body*, co-written with Vicki Edgson in 1999, has sold more than 1 million copies and been translated into nine languages. Ian subsequently wrote *The Food Doctor in the City* and *In Bed with The Food Doctor*. In 2003, *The Food Doctor Diet* became an instant bestseller and was tested on Channel 4's *Richard and Judy* by three volunteers, who each lost a dress size in only three weeks. Richard and Judy tested Ian's subsequent book, *The Food Doctor Everyday Diet* on six new volunteers over ten weeks, who all achieved similar results. *The Food Doctor Diet* has been hailed as a truly sensible, healthy approach to weight loss that really works.

The Food Doctor Everyday Diet plan

Ian Marber's Everyday Diet weight loss plan is designed to help those people unable to visit Ian for a personal consultation to rebalance their body systems and lose weight healthily and for the long term. The answer lies in identifying your metabolic rate, learning how to choose the right foods and, by doing so, rebalancing your metabolism to increase energy levels, motivation and ultimately weight loss. Yo-yo dieting disrupts the metabolic rate, meaning that the next time you restrict what you eat you tend not to lose the weight you have regained. This is why the Everyday Diet is just that, a diet plan that becomes a way of life as you follow 10 simple principles.

Acknowledgments

To the founder members of The Food Doctor Diet Club for their enthusiasm and willingness, and for their confidence in me and my plan. To everyone at The Food Doctor for their hard work and help, especially Michael da Costa and my wonderful assistant, Erika Andersson, for her constant care and patience. To Susannah Steel for her cheeriness and dedication, and to everyone at DK, especially Mary-Clare, Penny, Shannon, Catherine, Hermione and Antonia. To my friends at Cactus for their support, especially Amanda, Simon, Richard and Judy. The publisher would like to thank Hilary Bird for supplying the index and Ann Baggaley for proofreading.

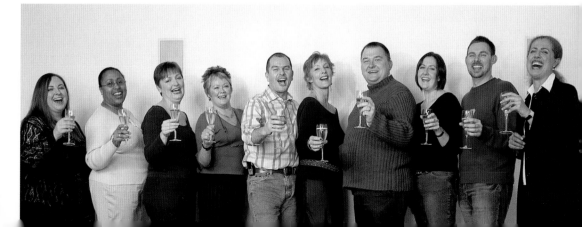

FOOD™ DOCTOR Think **Goodness** and change the **way** you eat **for Good** on us!

Let us help you with vouchers worth £50 redeemable against our range of foods, subscription web service, and even signing up to our Everyday Diet Weight Loss Plan. You can also save 15% on all DK titles

- **The Food Doctor, Ian Marber, with his team of nutrition experts,** has created a growing range of foods to help you make those healthier food choices that could make a difference to your general health and well-being. These are widely available in the UK's major multiples and independent retail food and health stores.

  Each is designed to help promote a healthier way of eating by encouraging the addition of fibre-rich foods, essential omega fats and protein to your daily intake. This helps balance blood sugar and puts you more in control of your diet.

  You will be able to redeem your vouchers worth £20 on **The Food Doctor** products at your local shop, where available, and enjoy what we have to offer.

- Our **new subscription web-based support service** will provide you with a constant source of nutritional information, delicious recipes and the inspiration to follow a healthier lifestyle – a FREE 30-day introductory offer worth £16.95 is available to you having purchased The Food Doctor Diet Club book.

- **Save 15% on DK books.** Visit www.dk.com to save 15% on all DK books, including all **The Food Doctor Diet** books. Just choose your books, enter the code FoodDr in the shopping basket coupon box and you'll save 15%! (Offer ends 1 January 2008).

- We can also help you follow a healthier balanced diet if you sign up to **The Food Doctor Everyday Diet Weight Loss Plan** at a discount of £12.50 (usual price £99).

To obtain your book of vouchers all you have to do is send a stamped addressed envelope with proof of purchase for this book along with your name and address to:

The Food Doctor Clinic, 76-78, Holland Park Avenue, London W11 3RB

Terms & Conditions: 1. Only available in the UK. 2. Please allow 14 days for delivery. 3. Closing date for receipt of applications for The Food Doctor book of redeemable vouchers worth £50 is 31st December 2007 4. No refund value is available on any vouchers, nor on the products or services provided. 5. No responsibility can be accepted for applications lost, delayed or damaged in the post – proof of posting is no proof of delivery. 6. Receipt for purchase of The Food Doctor Diet Club must be included with the application for vouchers. 7. We reserve the right to change the content of the offer at any time. Registered Office: The Food Doctor Limited as above.